Making the Time

An Expert Guide to Cross Country Riding

Stuart Tinney
Gold Medallist
Sydney Olympics
OAM

with

Alison Duthie

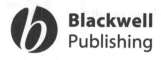
Blackwell
Publishing

Editorial Offices:
Blackwell Publishing Ltd, 9600 Garsington Road, Oxford OX4 2DQ, UK
    Tel: +44 (0)1865 776868
Blackwell Publishing Professional, 2121 State Avenue, Ames, Iowa 50014-8300,
USA
    Tel: +1 515 292 0140
Blackwell Publishing Asia Pty Ltd, 550 Swanston Street, Carlton, Victoria 3053,
Australia
    Tel: +61 (0)3 8359 1011

First published 2004 by Blackwell Publishing Ltd

Library of Congress Cataloging-in-Publication Data
is available

ISBN 1-4051-0292-6

A catalogue record for this title is available from the British Library

Set in 10/13 pt Palatino
by Graphicraft Limited, Hong Kong

The publisher's policy is to use permanent paper from mills that operate a
sustainable forestry policy, and which has been manufactured from pulp
processed using acid-free and elementary chlorine-free practices. Furthermore,
the publisher ensures that the text paper and cover board used have met
acceptable environmental accreditation standards.

For further information on Blackwell Publishing, visit our website:
www.blackwellpublishing.com

Contents

Foreword

I have always been impressed with Stuart Tinney as a rider, and when Stuart came to train with me, early on in his professional career, I quickly came to realise that not only could this young man ride but he was, and is, the ultimate perfectionist in everything he does with his horses. When I first started helping Stuart he could always see a stride into a fence – it just wasn't the best stride so we worked on changing it. For some it might take a lifetime, for Stuart it took 2 weeks of seriously hard work where he worked tirelessly on getting it right, falling off on several occasions in the process. But after 2 weeks Stuart had got it, and from then on he has never looked back. He takes his riding seriously, he thinks about his cross country riding every step of the way and never leaves anything to chance. He jumps each fence as it needs to be jumped, which goes a long way to making his cross country rounds as safe as they can possibly be. It is rare to see Stuart jump a fence badly, regardless of whether he is on his top horse or a youngster.

Stuart is also the master of timing. He will never push his horses more than necessary, believing that if you have walked the course correctly and if your horse has been trained correctly you will know how fast to go between fences to make the time. I'm delighted that Stuart has put his thoughts on cross country riding into a book and I feel confident that every reader will gain valuable insight into how to ride a safe cross country round while still making the time.

Wayne Roycroft
Chairman of the FEI Eventing Committee

Introduction

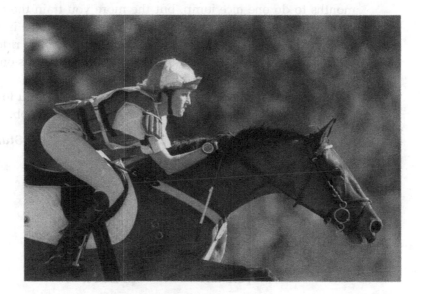

I decided to write this book because I wanted to help riders enjoy the sport I love. To enjoy eventing you must be able to ride in a safe way, and to ride in a safe way you must train your horse correctly. As you train your horse he will start to feel more confident in what he is doing, and consequently he will also start to enjoy his eventing.

Whether it is the thrill of galloping across the country or jumping fences out in the open, or simply just the horse and rider having a good time, it is the cross country phase of eventing that is the most popular with riders. It is also the phase with the greatest element of risk. Most riders spend hours training in the arena perfecting their dressage and show-jumping skills but cross country skills can sometimes be over-looked, and often the only practice the rider gets over cross country fences is at the event itself. Early on in the season eventing clinics are usually held, and I would advise all riders to attend as many of these as possible, but once the season begins many riders are left to their own devices. It is therefore essential to have some kind of idea of what to expect as different situations arise and also an idea of how to deal with them. That is what I hope to bring to you in this book. Most cross country riders want to be competitive and therefore they must learn how to both ride safely and make the time.

Although teaching your horse and yourself how to ride a cross country course safely takes time, patience and perseverance, the outcome will be well worth it. When you start your training it may take you months to do one nice jump, but the more you train the more often it will happen. That great feeling you get when a horse is going well makes all the hours of work worthwhile. The better you ride the more your horse will enjoy his eventing. Just look at the photos on these two pages – the horses look keen and focused on their job.

I hope you enjoy reading this book and if it helps you to ride more cross country rounds in a safer way it will have done its job.

Stuart Tinney

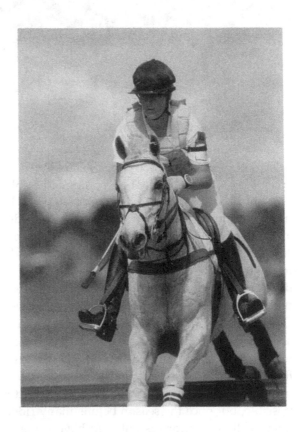

Acknowledgements

I would like to thank all the people who allowed me to achieve my dreams and who helped me to have my career with horses: Brian Tinney for all your support, Gwen Tinney, Colleen Fearnley, the late John Fearnley, the Stocker family, Vicky Roycroft and Wayne Roycroft for all you have taught me – thank you.

A special thank you to Alison Duthie for all her time and input in preparing this book, Max Wilson: Agenda Photography for his photography, and my family, Karen, Jaymee and Gemma.

Equipment for the horse and rider

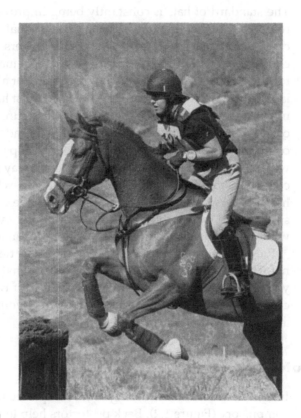

Figure 1.1

All riding activities, but particularly cross country, can be high risk, so it is important to make our riding as safe as we possibly can by using the safest equipment for both our horses and ourselves. Some equipment for the rider, such as hats and back protectors, have to be of a regulation standard, so contact your own Equestrian Federation for the current regulations. Whether it is equipment for yourself or your horse it must be both practical and comfortable to wear. The last thing you want to be thinking about as you go cross country is 'my new boots are cutting into the back of my knee', and the same goes for your horse.

EQUIPMENT FOR THE RIDER

Hat

The standard of hats is constantly being improved as more and more research is carried out into head injuries, so make sure when you purchase a hat that it meets current standards. Riders in hot climates should choose a hat with some ventilation as this will make the hat more comfortable to wear and keep you a little cooler. For all jumping, whether it is showjumping or cross country, your hat must have a chin strap and it must be securely fastened (Figure 1.1). Make sure the hat fits your head correctly. If it is too tight it could give you a headache, if it is too loose it could move around too much. A hat which slips around on your head will not only distract you when you ride but may not protect your head correctly should you fall. The choice of a silk, which is fitted over the hat, is a personal one. Some riders like to have colour coordinated hat silk, jumper, back protector, saddle cloth and even the horse's boots, while other riders are quite happy to settle for smart and tidy.

Riders with long hair should have it securely tied back or wear a hairnet. There are two reasons for this. The first is that if hair is constantly in your eyes you will find it hard to focus on your riding and, second, the cross country jump judges must be able to see your back number clearly and long, flapping hair will obscure their view.

Back protector

In most countries the wearing of a back protector for cross country is compulsory (Figure 1.2). Back protectors help to protect the rider from penetrating injuries (for example, landing on rocks) and they will also soften the blow of a fall. Imagine the difference between falling off onto concrete and falling off onto sand – which would you choose?

It is important to try on several types of back protector until you find one which is comfortable for you and will not interfere with your position as you ride. Although a back protector may seem quite an expensive outlay they are usually adjustable to various sizes, making it

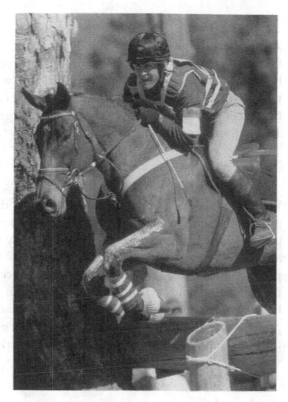

Figure 1.2   This rider is using a Dutch gag with one rein, a Hanoverian noseband and an elastic stockman's breastplate with a running martingale attachment; he is wearing his back protector, medical armband and gloves.

something that a child will not grow out of in 6 months and that an adult should be able to use for several years. Depending on the type of back protector you choose it can be worn under or over your jumper or cross country shirt.

Boots

Riding boots, whether they are rubber or leather, must be in good repair and it is very important that the sole is in one piece. A flapping sole can get caught in the stirrup, which could interfere with the way you ride or at worst could lead to a fall. The boots should be a good fit for your feet and a good fit in the stirrup. As a guide you should be able to fit one finger-width either side of your foot when it is in the stirrup. If the boots are too big or the stirrups too small your foot could easily be caught in the stirrup should you fall.

Spurs

Although spurs are not actually a safety equipment item, it is important that they are fitted correctly. When you put on your spurs make sure the buckle is done up on the outside of your boot, with the end strap pointing downwards and towards the back of your boot. If the buckle sits at the top of your boot there is a chance it could get caught on the stirrup and, in the event of a fall, this could lead to your foot getting trapped.

Gloves

Wearing gloves is a personal choice, but you do need to have a good grip on the reins at all times and for this reason many riders consider gloves to be an essential item for cross country (Figure 1.2). When you are choosing gloves try to imagine that you will be saturated at some point on the course. This could be from the weather conditions, a fall into water or simply from cantering through water, but however it happens you still need to have a good grip on the reins. For that reason I prefer not to use leather gloves as I find they get quite slippery when they are wet, so I go for gloves which will work equally well in dry or wet conditions.

Medical armband

It is compulsory at all official one-day and three-day events for competitors to wear medical armbands. These can usually be purchased from your Equestrian Federation or from saddleries. The armband contains a card on which are all your medical details, vital information for the paramedics or doctors should you suffer a fall. Make sure all your details are correct, up to date and written clearly. The medical armband must be carried visibly either on your arm (Figure 1.2) or attached to your back protector. Some countries specify where the medical armbands should be worn, so check with your Equestrian Federation.

Watch

A watch could be classed as a piece of safety equipment as it will help you to go at the correct speed on a cross country course. I use a watch at all levels of eventing so I never have to gallop my horses harder than necessary to make the time. Wearing a watch takes away the 'guess' element when you are going cross country, and it will also help to stop you making those irritating mistakes such as coming in two seconds

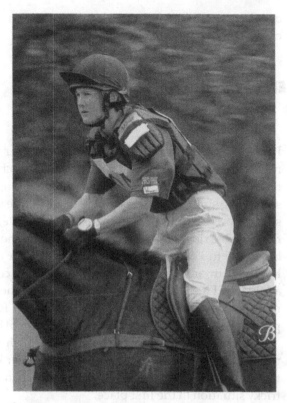

Figure 1.3   This rider is using an elastic chest breastplate on her horse and is riding in a flat saddle with a saddlecloth and pad. She is wearing her medical armband on the shoulder pad of her back protector; her watch is clearly visible on her wrist.

over time and losing the event. Riders who choose not to wear watches may think they are not going fast enough and will speed up, perhaps unnecessarily.

Use a watch with an easy to read face (Figure 1.3) as you need to be able to look at it and instantly see if you have to speed up or slow down. Watches that have a beeping mechanism are particularly useful at three-day events as you can set them to beep every minute, helping you to judge if you are up to or behind the minute markers on the course. (Minute markers are explained in Chapter 2.)

Other clothing

The type of jodhpurs, breeches, shirts or jumpers worn for cross country are a personal preference. Some people like to wear a stock, not just for dressage and showjumping, but for cross country as well. If you do decide to do this make sure you don't wear a stock pin as this could cause a problem if you have a fall.

EQUIPMENT FOR THE HORSE

Saddle

I prefer to ride in a flat-seated saddle, in other words a saddle with a relatively low cantle. Any saddle with too much of a cantle can tend to hit you in the bottom, especially if you are going down a drop fence or something similar, whereas a flat-seated saddle will allow you to be in a strong position but not held there by the saddle, which I like. Very few falls involve riders falling off backwards and therefore you don't need a big cantle to keep you in. In addition, I prefer a saddle which doesn't hold you in any one place because in cross country you need to be adaptable. I also find that using a flat saddle helps you create a better, more independent position because it won't force you into a certain position and you start to find your own point of balance.

Knee rolls on jumping saddles are very much a personal choice. Some riders like the feeling of being able to jam their knees into something if they are in a tricky situation. Of course, it is better to avoid being in that tricky situation in the first place.

The saddle must fit the horse and the rider so don't buy a saddle until you have tried it on your horse and ridden in it. It could be completely unsuitable for the type of horse you have and it may not fit your body shape. Check there is good clearance off the horse's back through the gullet of the saddle. This can be a problem with some of the new flat saddles, especially if they are used on high withered horses. The Bates 'Cair' range of saddles and other 'air' saddles suit most horses as they rely on air pillows as their cushioning. The other good point about these saddles is that they have changeable gullets, which can be very handy when you have to use one saddle for more than one horse as it makes fitting the saddle to each horse relatively simple.

Saddlecloths and pads

The saddlecloth must fit the saddle you are using. If it is too small the saddle will stick out beyond the saddlecloth which could lead to a sore spot on the horse's back, or at the very least the horse's coat will be rubbed. If the saddlecloth is too big it will cover up too much of the horse's cooling system – his skin – and this can make a big difference on a hot day. Sometimes the use of a pad is necessary, but take care that you don't add too much weight to the whole saddle. For this reason I use light foam pads or closed cell foam pads as they do the job without adding any significant weight.

Stirrups

Your stirrups must be the correct size for your feet and boots with clearance of a finger width on both sides. If you have a fall wearing stirrups which are the correct size, the chances are your feet will simply slip out of the stirrups. If the stirrups are too small there is a chance your foot could get stuck, which could result in you being dragged. Stirrups that are too big could allow your foot to slip right through, again raising the possibility of being dragged. I find aluminium stirrup irons the best as they are very light and if your foot slips out they are easy to find again as they don't tend to swing around too much. Stainless steel stirrup irons are another good choice, although they are much heavier than aluminium so they might not be your choice if you are trying to keep weight to a minimum. I would not recommend the use of nickel stirrup irons as they will not stand up to too much pressure and are more likely to break than the other two options.

Girths

I prefer to use girths with some amount of elastic in them. I believe these types of girth are more comfortable for the horse as they expand with him as he changes his body shape. It is vital the elastic is in good condition and not at all perished or worn, so keep a careful check for any signs of wear and tear. Girths that have been in storage for some time must be checked thoroughly before they are used as the elastic can perish from age. When fitting a girth of any description take care not to overtighten it as you may affect the horse's ability to breathe properly, or at the very least cause a pinch or a sore area. In the case of an elastic girth make sure the elastic still looks like elastic, with some give in it and not pulled to its limit.

Girth points

On your saddle you will see three girth points. Two of these points, usually the second and third, are connected to one strap and the other point has its own strap. All the straps go over the tree of the saddle. To be safe, when you do up your girth attach it to the points on different straps, that is, either the first and second or the first and third. By doing this, if one strap should break the girth will still be attached to the other strap.

Overgirth

An overgirth gives some added security as it will help to keep your saddle in place should your girth break. I don't use an overgirth at one-day events, but I do make sure my girths and girth points are in excellent condition. When fitting, the buckle of the overgirth should sit under the horse's belly so that it will not interfere with the rider's leg or hit the horse's elbow as he gallops. If you do choose to wear an overgirth take care that, like the girth, it is not done up too tightly and that it sits neatly on top of your normal girth. An overgirth which slips back and sits behind the girth can badly pinch the horse's skin.

Breastplate

A correctly fitted breastplate will prevent the saddle from slipping backwards and they are commonly used by many riders when going cross country. When fitting the breastplate it should look slightly loose when the horse is standing still. The slack will be taken up as the horse jumps a fence (Figure 1.4). If a breastplate is fitted too tightly it may restrict the jumping action of the horse. I prefer to use a stockman's breastplate, with elastic, as I feel it allows the horse plenty of freedom when jumping.

Martingale

A martingale is not so much a piece of safety equipment as a piece of training equipment, so before you automatically reach for a martingale ask yourself the question, 'Does my horse need a martingale?' Some horses will definitely not improve with the addition of a martingale and it can have a detrimental effect, so you must be sure why you are using it. Ask your instructor for advice and make sure you try out the martingale at home before you use it at an event.

A running martingale should be fitted so that the rings of the martingale go up to the gullet of the horse when he is standing in a natural position. Another way to check the fitting is to put the martingale on the horse and adjust it so that the rings stretch from the centre of the chest to the withers. If the martingale is fitted correctly the steering of the horse should not be affected and the martingale will only come into play after the horse has put his head up quite high. If your reins have buckles where

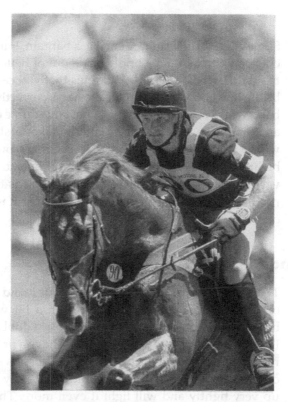

Figure 1.4   In this photograph we can see a Dutch gag (the same bit as shown in Figure 1.2) being used, but in this instance the rider has chosen to use it with an equaliser attached to the top and bottom ring. A grakle noseband is also being used together with two elastic breastplates, a stockman's and a chest one. The rider is wearing all his safety equipment including hat, back protector, medical armband, watch and gloves.

they attach onto the bit, make sure you fit rubber stoppers on the reins to prevent the rings of the martingale getting caught in the buckles.

Reins

I prefer to use rubber reins for both showjumping and cross country, but it is really an individual choice and many people prefer to ride with webbing reins. Whatever your choice, you must be able to hold the reins whether they are wet or dry. Like all tack you must be sure your reins are in good order. It is difficult to know the condition of the leather underneath rubber reins, so replace them on a regular basis. I tend to use reins which have looped ends instead of buckles as I find they are less likely to break and it also means you don't have to worry about the rings of a martingale getting caught in the buckles.

Bridle

Some cheap bridles may seem like a bargain, but they are more prone to crack and break than a bridle made out of better quality leather, so try to invest in the best bridle and reins that you can afford. Make sure the bridle is in good order and fits the horse correctly. For example, a browband which is too big must be a constant source of irritation to the horse as it bangs on his head each time he takes a step, while a throat lash which is too tight may restrict the horse's outline and possibly his breathing. One of the most important things to remember when using various pieces of equipment on your horse is to use what your horse needs and not to just use something because it is in fashion and 'everyone' is using it.

Nosebands

There are various types of noseband, but I tend to stick to the common ones. I use a cavesson noseband with a bit which doesn't need the bottom strap of a noseband (for example, a double bridle), but generally I use a Hanoverian noseband. Unless I have a problem with a horse who really wants to open his mouth I fit nosebands so they are firm but not overtight. Some horses may become irritated by a noseband that is done up very tightly and will fight it even more. The choice of nosebands, as with a lot of other equipment, comes down to what your horse is comfortable with and what he works best in.

Boots and bandages

Whether you choose to use boots or bandages on your horse's legs when you go cross country, they must do two things:

(1) Protect without rubbing
(2) Not absorb water.

Protection without rubbing

The horse's legs must be protected from injury which could be caused by a blow from another leg or from hitting a fence. On the front leg the most important area to protect is the back of the leg where the major tendons and ligaments are situated. This area can be seriously injured if the back legs come through to the front legs before the front legs are out of the way. The front of the front leg should, hopefully, not hit too many fences, so it has a minimal risk of being injured. On the back leg it is the other way around. The front of the leg needs protection from scraping over or hitting a fence, whereas the back of the leg should be relatively safe from any injury, unless it scrapes down a drop fence or something similar.

Some boots will rub the horse's leg, which can be very painful for the horse and can often be the cause of horses failing the trot-up on Sunday morning. If you find that your horse's boots are rubbing, put a small amount of talcum powder down the inside of the boot as this usually helps to lessen the problem. If the problem persists, change to a new type of boot with a softer lining.

Water absorption

It is no help to your horse if you use a boot or bandage which soaks up water as this will only make the legs heavier for the horse to carry. It could also cause the horse to be slower in galloping or picking his legs up, which could lead to over-reaching.

I prefer to use 'porter boots' for cross country. They are made of high density foam and wrap around the horse's leg. The porter boot has several advantages over other materials, one being that you can cut the boot to fit each individual horse and it is very strong and will withstand a blow. Porter boots do not have any fastening, so for one-day events I use an outer covering wrap of leather with buckles and for three-day events I bandage over the porter boots using a self-sticking bandage such as Vetwrap. I finish off by securing the bandage with some eventing tape.

Fitting boots and bandages

The boots on the front legs must not be fitted too high or they will inter-fere with the action of the horse's knee which, in turn, may affect his jumping ability. To ensure the boots aren't too high after you have fitted them pick up the horse's leg and bend it at the knee to check that the top of the boot doesn't dig into the back of the knee joint. Back boots must also cover as much of the leg as possible without interfering with his action so after you have fitted the back boots, walk and trot the horse in hand.

Boots and bandages must be fitted with even pressure to avoid damage to any part of the leg. When putting on bandages do not pull the bandage too tight. If you are unsure of the firmness required for band-ages ask your instructor. When fitting boots, do up the middle buckle or Velcro strap first, followed by the bottom and top, as this will help to keep the pressure even.

Bell or over-reach boots

Bell or over-reach boots protect the heels on the front foot from injury. Over-reaching is caused by the toe of the back shoe catching the bulbs of the heel on the front foot. Many over-reaching problems can be helped, to a great extent, by a good farrier and corrective shoeing. Slowing down the back feet a little and speeding up the front feet by rolling the toes can stop a horse over-reaching, but some horses, despite the best efforts of the farrier, will still catch themselves when galloping or jumping. Some riders use over-reach boots as a matter of course, but I don't like to use them unless I know a horse has this particular problem.

The cheapest, most common bell boots are made of rubber, but these boots do seem to cause more falls than bell boots made of other materials. When a horse jumps into water the drag of the water on the rubber will cause him to take slightly longer to get his front feet out of the way of his back feet and in this situation the horse can step on the boots and fall. Bell boots made of dense foam or leather do not seem to have such an effect as they tend to cut or break. Another choice is to use bell boots made of individual plastic petals. These boots work well because if the horse catches a boot, a petal breaks away so the horse is less likely to fall. However, I find, and I'm sure the horse would agree, that the noise of the flapping petals as you gallop along is really distracting and for that reason I don't use them.

Grease

Eventing grease is used, in theory, to help the horse slide over a fence if he should hit it. I'm not 100% convinced of that theory, but I am sure that using too much grease blocks up the horse's cooling system – his skin – and he is then not able to cool down quickly. For that reason I keep the use of grease to a minimum and only apply it to the horse's stifles which is an area commonly caught on a fence. Great care must be taken when applying grease as it can be dangerous if it ends up on the rider's boots, reins or another vital piece of equipment.

Studs

If your horse is not particularly well balanced or the going is slippery, the use of studs will give him a little more confidence. It is pointless to use studs in very heavy, deep going as they will have little, if any, effect; at the other extreme, if the ground is very hard, studs will only help to jar the horse's legs. However, using studs on ground which is firm but a bit slippery can certainly help, as the studs will grip the corners a little more, giving the horse confidence that he will not slip. Care must be taken not to over-stud a horse, in other words to use bigger studs than necessary. This is especially relevant at a three-day event where the roads and tracks could involve many kilometres of trotting on hard ground before the cross country course is reached. In this situation use very small studs, if any, as you set off on phase A, and wait until you come into the ten-minute box to change into bigger studs if you still feel you need them. That way you will not jar the horse more than necessary and yet have the grip you require for cross country. I like to keep the horse's foot even by putting two studs in each foot. If the horse's foot hits the ground evenly you are less likely to do damage to joints. When using studs, bear in mind how your horse jumps. If he is very neat and really tucks his front legs up you may find the studs will cut into him just behind the girth. Using a belly guard attached onto your girth will help to protect that area.

Bits

When you are going cross country, it is vital to be in control of your horse. To enable you to be in control you must train the horse correctly so he will listen to your aids to increase speed or slow down. The type of bit you choose to use for cross country should give you this control. I prefer to use snaffle bits, but I will move up to a stronger bit if I think it is necessary.

When you work your horse in the arena you will get an idea of how strong he is on the flat and over showjumps. If you take him out in an open paddock for some gallop work you might find he becomes a little stronger, or he could just stay the same as he was in the arena, but it is not until you take him on the cross country course that you will discover what he is like to ride when you are galloping, rebalancing, jumping and galloping again.

I tend to categorise bits into four groups:

(1) Snaffles
(2) Curbs – Pelhams/Kimblewicks (double bridles are a combination of a snaffle bit and a curb)
(3) Gags
(4) Hackamores

It is difficult to say that a certain bit will have the same effect on all horses. I have found some softer bits have a strong reaction with some horses, and equally strong bits can have no effect on other horses. Because of this, finding the right bit for each horse can be a matter of trial and error, but I would advise that you keep your search as simple as possible.

Snaffles

The basic bit is an eggbutt snaffle (Figure 1.5, right), and this is what I would usually use on a horse when I first start off. The same bit with a loose ring connection may be useful for a horse which doesn't turn easily as the loose ring tends to be a bit sharper, that is, it tends to have more of a reaction. If you want to move into something a notch stronger than a normal eggbutt snaffle, try a thinner snaffle like a racing D. The thinner mouthpiece makes the bit sharper and the bar connection at the end of the mouthpiece can help in turning. On the other hand, some horses who tend to lean can sometimes lean even more on the bar, so a loose ring snaffle (Figure 1.5, left) may be a better option for that type of horse.

One move up from a thinner snaffle could include a Dr Bristol (Figure 1.6, middle), a French link (Figure 1.5, middle), a twisted snaffle

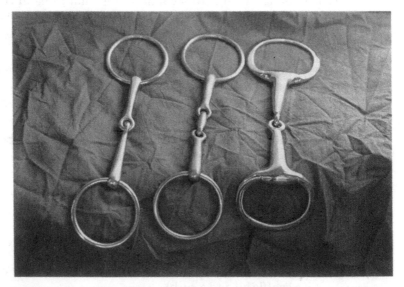

Figure 1.5   Left: A loose ring medium thickness snaffle, which could be used to start a horse off in – the loose ring may help when you're turning the horse. Middle: A loose ring French link snaffle – usually a little stronger than a thinner snaffle, but not with all horses. Right: A thick eggbutt snaffle, which could be used on a 'normal' horse, that is one who doesn't pull too much – be careful that the thickness of the bit doesn't overstretch and split the skin around the sides of the mouth.

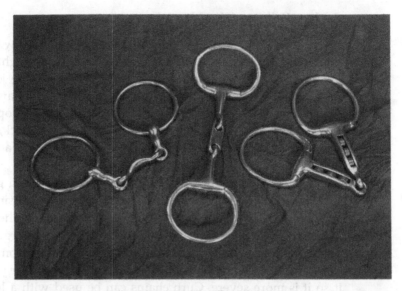

Figure 1.6   Left: A loose ring French link snaffle with port – a port in a mouthpiece can work quite well for some horses as it allows more room for the tongue and can also act on the roof of the horse's mouth. Middle: An eggbutt Dr Bristol – the angled plate should make the bit stronger than a French link. Right: A Mcguinness – the rollers in the mouthpiece can have a shock value for the horse and he will be less inclined to lock onto the bit.

or a W mouth bit. I have used the W bit with some success. I don't consider it to be a strong bit, but it does seem to have a shock value to the horse because it basically has two mouthpieces, which most horses aren't used to. The horse is also less likely to lock onto a bit with two mouthpieces. French link snaffles, which have a different shaped link in the centre of an otherwise normal snaffle, seem to be softer on some horses and stronger on others, so again it is a case of seeing what works for your horse. Although they look very similar, I do find a difference between riding in a French link and a Dr Bristol. The Dr Bristol has a plate which sits in the centre of the bit at a 45 degree angle, and for most horses it is a little sharper than a French link snaffle. There are two ways of putting in a Dr Bristol: you can put it in so the plate sits angled forward or turned upside down so it is angled back.

Snaffles like the cherry roller or Mcguinness (Figure 1.6, right) can also fall into the shock value category. I don't find them to be strong bits, but because they have rollers either on the outside of the mouthpiece, as in the case of the cherry roller, or within the mouthpiece, as in the case of the Mcguinness, many horses don't want to lock on or lean on them.

Curbs – Pelhams/Kimblewicks

I have used Pelhams and Kimblewicks (sometimes known as Spanish snaffles) with some success on horses with dull, slightly ignorant mouths. They come in a variety of mouthpieces, some jointed some straight. I don't particularly like the straight bars, but I have found that straight bars with a port can work quite well as they stop the tongue going over the bit. The Pelham is similar to the Kimblewick, but because it has a longer shank it will have more leverage than a Kimblewick (Figure 1.7).

The addition of a curb chain to these types of bit can give you the sharper reaction you are looking for in a horse who sits on the bit and pulls. The good point about using a chain is that the majority of horses seem to find it fairly inoffensive and they won't argue too much. The curb chain can be fitted loose or tight, depending on your needs. You can also fit the chain so it lies flat against the jaw, or you can twist it so it is more severe. Curb chains can be used with a leather cover

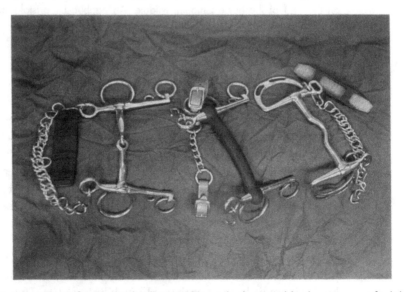

Figure 1.7   Left: A jointed Pelham with a curb chain and leather cover – I find the jointed Pelham has less lever action than a straight bar Pelham; the curb chain would be softened by the use of the leather cover. Middle: A vulcanite Pelham with curb chain – a vulcanite mouthpiece is usually thicker than a straight stainless steel mouthpiece so tends to be a little softer; however, I don't find the difference significant. Right: A Kimblewick or Spanish snaffle with a port and a curb chain with a rubber cover – a Kimblewick gives you the choice of attaching the rein to the top or bottom opening depending on the leverage you require.

to make them softer or, if you don't want to use a chain at all, you can substitute a rubber or gel pad which is attached in the same way as a curb chain (Figure 1.7).

Gags

Gags generally have a snaffle mouthpiece of some description, but they also work on a lever action which pulls down on the horse's poll. Because of this, gags can work quite well on horses who travel with a very high head carriage, or on horses who tend to throw their head in the air when you ask them to slow down. If you are riding a horse who has a low head carriage, or who bores down on the bit, a gag is possibly not the best option as it may make the problem worse. However, if the gag stops the horse leaning he might then travel in a better frame. It is a good idea to use cheekers when you are using gags, because the running action of the bit can pinch the sides of the horse's mouth.

Running gags have cheek straps made of leather or rope, which run through the rings of the bit. Basically speaking, a running gag (Figure 1.8, centre) will give you more pulling power. If you pull with a force of one kilogram a running gag will give you two kilograms. For this reason, you must be sure that a gag bit is required and that you will not pull your horse's mouth unnecessarily. Many horses have been put off jumping by riders who have pulled too hard in a strong bit while riding into and/or over a fence. If you are unsure about what sort of bit you need, ask your instructor or an experienced rider. When a bit works, that is when your horse has listened to your aids to slow down, make sure you trust the bit and allow the horse to travel along until you have to use the slowing down aids again. Make sure you don't pull on the bit and consequently the horse's mouth the whole time.

All bits must be fitted correctly so that they are comfortable for the horse. This is especially important in the case of gag bits if they are to have their desired effect. Dutch gags (Figure 1.8, right) have to be fitted very high in the horse's mouth so when you use the rein the lever action comes into play straight away. If they are fitted too low they will not work as they are meant to. As the Dutch gag has a curved shank I don't think it has a great gag action and doesn't seem to be as strong as an American gag (Figure 1.8, left), which has a longer straighter shank. I find a correctly fitted American gag the best bit to use on a very strong horse because its long shank gives it plenty of leverage yet it still gives you the use and steering of a snaffle mouthpiece.

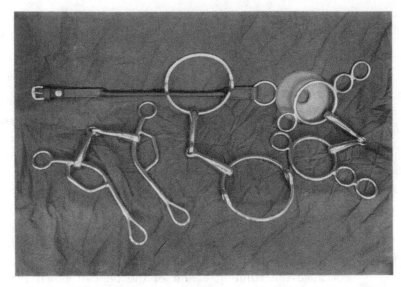

Figure 1.8   Left: A snaffle mouthed American gag – I find this the best type of bit to use on a strong horse; because of the length of the shank these bits have very good leverage. Middle: A running gag with snaffle mouthpiece – when the reins are used the bit will run the length of the leather cheek pieces. Right: A Dutch gag with snaffle mouthpiece and rubber cheekers – the cheek pieces attach onto the top ring and the reins can be attached to any of the next three rings, depending on the severity required; the rubber cheekers will help to prevent the sides of the horse's mouth being pinched as the bit slides up and down, and soaking them in hot water will make it easier to pull them over the ends of the bit. All the gag bits shown have snaffle mouthpieces so they will have a snaffle action as well as the gag action.

Riding in two reins

If possible, I try to avoid riding in two reins simply because it is easier to use one. However, if I do decide to ride in a Pelham or a double bridle I will use two reins. After galloping between fences I use more of the bottom rein, which is the stronger rein, to do my rebalancing, and once I am at the required speed I will ride over the fence with the top, softer rein. Some riders are concerned that they might not always know which rein they are using when they are jumping a combination fence, but if, for example, you jump into the water and lose your reins, I don't think it really matters which rein you gather up first. Even if there is another fence to jump in the water, the horse should still be under control as you will be in a steadier pace. The stronger rein should only become vital to use once you have galloped on after the fence and are coming towards your next point of rebalancing. In theory, you should use more of your bottom reins to slow down from gallop and more of the top rein through the fence.

Equalisers

When you use a bit like a Pelham or a Dutch gag or, in fact, any type of bit where you have a choice of different places to put the reins instead of using two reins, you can use an equaliser so that you only have to use one rein rather than two. However, you can find that in doing that you lose some of the lever action of the bit, because the equaliser won't allow you to use the strong bit fully. However, if your horse likes the combination of the two bits an equaliser can work quite well. If you look in Figures 1.2 and 1.4 you will see that the same bit is being used, but one rider has chosen to use an equaliser while the other rider just uses one rein.

Hackamore

Hackamores have the reputation of being quite strong, but I don't find that at all. They have no mouthpiece and they work from pressure on the nose and the jaw (from the chain) (Figure 1.9). Although they are not generally used by themselves for cross country they are sometimes used in conjunction with a bit, in which case you would be riding with two reins. In this scenario it would be similar to riding in a double bridle,

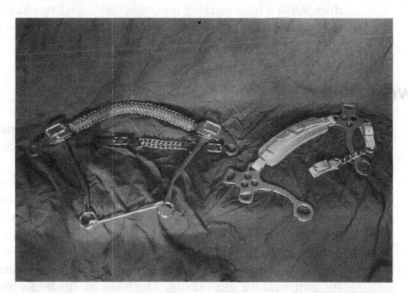

Figure 1.9 The longer the shank on the hackamore, or on any other bit, the stronger it will be, so the hackamore on the left would be the most severe. However, I don't find any hackamore to be that strong. Hackamores are not generally used by themselves for cross country, but they can be a useful alternative in the showjumping phase for a sensitive horse, or they can be used in conjunction with a bit for cross country.

only the bit rein would be your rebalancing rein and you would use more of the hackamore through the fences. Hackamores are really useful for horses who are very reactive to the bit no matter how soft it is, and they can also be useful if you have a horse with a cut mouth. For both of these reasons a hackamore might be your choice for showjumping. I find horses are the same in their body whether you ride them in a bit or a hackamore. For example, if your horse is stiff to the right when you ride him in a bit, he will still be stiff to the right when you ride him in a hackamore, because this is related to the suppleness of his body, it is not a bit problem.

Mouthpieces

Most bits come in a variety of mouthpieces and they also vary in their thickness. Generally a thicker mouthpiece will be softer than a thin one. A thin mouthpiece, if used too sharply, can cut the horse's mouth, but I have found that thick ones can do the same because they seem to overstretch and split the skin. Mouthpieces can be made from stainless steel, copper, sweet iron, vulcanite, rubber, plastic or a combination of several of these. If the horse is not salivating the bit, which he should, I don't believe changing the metal in the bit is the answer. The horse will produce saliva if he is working the correct way, so if you have a problem in this area do some more training on the flat and make the horse use his jaw a little more.

WEAR AND TEAR

One of the most important things you can do for your own safety is to keep a good check on all the tack you use on your horse. Some areas are more prone to stress than others, so get into the habit of looking at each individual piece for signs of wear and tear. Common places likely to get worn are the cheek pieces and the reins where they attach onto the bit, and the bit itself. Metal fatigue is not always easy to spot, but you can see if your bit is wearing in one area, possibly the connection in the middle of the bit, and if this is happening replace the bit. Stress areas on the saddle include where the stirrup irons sit on the stirrup leathers, the girth and the girth points. The holes on the bridle and saddle, for example the holes on the girth points, are under a lot of pressure and also need to be checked regularly to make sure they are not starting to rip. Also keep a check on the stitching on your reins, stirrup leathers and all stitching on the saddle and bridle.

TROUBLESHOOTING

Q: My horse bores down and gets very heavy when I ride him cross country. What should I do?
Sometimes boring down is just the way the horse gallops naturally, so all you can do is make sure he will listen to your rebalancing aids when you are approaching a fence. It is just like riding on the flat. If you were trotting in the arena and your horse started to get heavy and go on the forehand you would half halt, perhaps several times, to tell him to pick up his forehand and withers and travel in a better way. Relate that to cross country. Firstly, you must have a sharp enough bit so he will respond to you. Secondly, give him the half halt aid until he responds. He might only travel in the frame you want for a short time, and if that was the case you would give him the half halt aid again to recorrect him. It is important that you don't just lean or pull on the horse the whole time, because this will make it harder to rebalance him and you might also cut his mouth. The other option is to allow the horse to travel the way he wants to on the cross country course, having the confidence that you will be able to adjust his frame and rebalance before the next fence. You do not want to jump a fence with a horse who is travelling in a very flat frame, as he will be more likely to hit the fence.

Don't hang onto the horse's mouth after you have rebalanced him as this will only make him lean more

Q: Do you try out new bits at home before using them at an event? And what bit should I start with?
I find it hard to emulate cross country anywhere else other than on a cross country course in competition, so although I might try out a new bit at home I won't expect to get the same feeling as I will when I'm out on the cross country course. I generally start horses off in a normal snaffle, that is, a snaffle with a medium thickness mouthpiece. After I have ridden cross country I will assess how the horse felt and make a decision regarding which bit to use for the next event. I tend to work on the following:

- Sensible to ride – stick to the same bit
- A little strong – thinner snaffle
- Quite strong – Dr Bristol or similar
- Dull or ignorant in the mouth – Kimblewick or Pelham
- Very strong – some sort of gag

I usually find that horses only need one change of bit. For example, if I start them in a fat snaffle I might move to a thin snaffle and they will generally then stay in that bit. If the horse has been trained correctly, I shouldn't find it necessary to move up to a stronger bit as he moves up the levels of eventing.

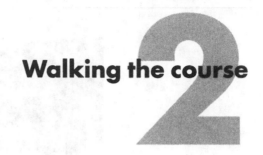

Walking the course

WHY DO YOU NEED TO WALK THE COURSE?

Walking the cross country course gives you an opportunity to look at all the fences your horse will have to jump and the terrain he will have to negotiate. Your horse doesn't get the same opportunity, so you must gather sufficient information from walking the course to then be able to pass it on to your horse as you ride around the course. For example, your horse won't know there is a difficult combination fence around the next corner, but you will, so you must rebalance and ride in a way that will allow him to make the best possible effort over that fence. There is usually enough time at a one-day event to walk the course twice. The first time gives you a chance to get an overall feel of what the course is like, and many riders will do this first walk with some friends (Figure 2.1); however, the second course walk is much more serious as it is then that you have to make decisions about the lines you will ride and how you will jump each fence. You can walk the course as many times as you want to, and certainly at a three-day event most riders walk the course at least three times. Try to take one of your walks with either an experienced rider or your instructor. Most experienced riders are only too happy to be asked for their opinion. At some bigger events there are often course walks, organised by the event committee, taken by an elite rider. Even if you are just spectating at an event where this is available, join in and take advantage of it, as you could learn some useful tips which could help you with your own eventing.

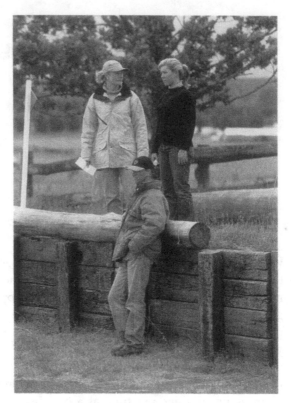

Figure 2.1 Riders assessing a fence during a course walk.

CHOICES

As I said, the advice of an experienced rider can be very helpful because courses are becoming more and more technical, so you must walk the course with some knowledge of what the course designer is asking you to do. For example, he may have built a combination of two fences with a distance of two long strides between them. It is up to you to realise that the distance is long and ride the fence accordingly. Each fence will dictate what speed it should be jumped at, and to jump it safely you must jump it at that speed. Of course, if you jump it faster than required you might get away with it, but it could unsettle your horse for the next jump. The speed at which you decide to jump each fence is your choice, but you are taking a risk if you jump fences faster than necessary. For this reason I will jump each fence at the speed it dictates, and then gallop safely at whatever speed I need to make up the time. For example, if I am riding a course which has a speed of 550 metres/minute and I have jumped some fences at 350 metres/minute, I know that somewhere on the course I will have to gallop at 700 metres/minute to make up the time. If the course is hilly and twisty, the time will usually be much harder to make up than on, say, a flatter, straighter course. As you walk the course be aware of the areas that will allow you to make up time. Whatever speed you choose to ride at, you must ride safely, because it will not help if you slip or fall through galloping too fast round a tight corner in an effort to make up time.

CONDITIONS

When you walk the course, take note of the ground conditions. If it is raining in the morning and you're not riding until the afternoon, the ground might deteriorate during the day, so ask yourself, 'Are there places on the course which are or could get slippery?' This could be relevant when you are travelling round a corner, and bear in mind that even hard ground can be slippery. Take particular notice of the light and shadows, especially if you will be jumping from light to dark or dark to light. Sometimes the position of the sun and the shadows can play a big part in how a fence might look to a horse and how he judges it. In Australia we don't jump a lot of fences going from light to dark, but we may be asked to jump a fence in the shade of a tree. If you have to jump a fence like this you must give the horse enough time to focus on what he has to do.

WORKING OUT WHERE YOU SHOULD BE AT WHAT TIME

If you want to make the time on the cross country phase, you must know if you are behind or up on time as you travel around the course. For a one-day event which has a relatively short cross country track, it is not really feasible to work out minute markers, but it is possible to work out where a rough half-way point is on the course, which will certainly be of some help. Although using a measuring wheel is by far the most accurate way of measuring a course, most people, certainly at a one-day event, don't have access to a wheel, so the following can act as a guide. As you set off on one of your course walks take note of the time. For this exercise to work you must walk consistently around the track; in other words, don't stop for a chat half-way round. Take note of the time when you finish your walk. Let's imagine it has taken you 50 minutes to walk the whole course. When you walk the course again, repeat the exercise knowing that 25 minutes into your walk will roughly be the half-way point. If the first half of the course is very hilly and the second part is flat you will usually be able to make up time on the flat section, so it won't matter too much if you reach your half-way point a little behind the clock.

Minute markers

At a three-day event you will need to be much more accurate. Using a measuring wheel, walk the course, and you should find that your measurements agree with those of the course designers. Know what your set speed is for the level you are riding; for example, 530 metres/minute for a novice three-day event. In other words, each 530 metres on the course should take 1 minute. As you walk the course with your wheel, note when the wheel reads 530 metres and this will be your first minute marker; your second minute marker will be when the wheel reads 1060 metres and the third will be when it reads 1590 metres. This will continue through to the end of the course.

Working out your time for a three-day event

When you are at a three-day event, you have to know your times for riding all four phases of the speed and endurance day so that you can come in under time and avoid any penalties. Most riders write the information they need on their arm where it can be seen quickly and easily, but not all riders write the same information. Personally I don't like to write down too much. I will know that the times at the top refer to phase A and the next line refers to phase B, so I simply write down my start and finish time for phases A, B and C and the optimum time for those phases. For phase D, I write only the start time because the time for phase D and the minute markers will all be in my head. At the start of phase D, I simply start my watch from zero and will know that I have to be through the finish when it is reading the optimum time if I am to avoid any penalties. The information on my arm would look something like Figure 2.2.

	START	FINISH	TIME
A	11.47	12.07	20
B	12.08	12.11	3
C	12.11	12.56	45
D	1.06		9.47

Figure 2.2

KNOWING AT WHAT SPEED TO TRAVEL

Before you ride in your first three-day event you will be well practised, from your one-day events, at judging the speed you have to travel in order to make time on the cross country course. You will jump each fence at the speed it dictates and ride accordingly in between the fences to come in at the correct time. However, it is not until you come to ride at a three-day event that you will need to know what pace is required in the roads and tracks phase. For example, let's say phase A is 4400 metres long and has to be ridden in 20 minutes. If you take 4 minutes to cover each kilometre you will take 17 minutes 36 seconds to ride 4400 metres. This is where judgement comes into play. There is no point arriving too early at the next phase, so this speed of a kilometre every 4 minutes would allow you to walk at some stage on phase A. As phase A is a warm-up phase, you might decide to give your horse some consistent trotting and possibly a short canter to get him ready for the steeplechase phase. Because of this, it would be a good idea to walk towards the end of phase A so that your horse is settled down before phase B. Of course, each horse is different, and you must do whatever works for your horse; this may mean walking in the middle of phase A and trotting at the end. I try to plan on getting to the end of phase A around 30 seconds early, which will allow for anything going wrong; for example, a boot might need to be adjusted.

Phase C is a recovery phase and is therefore treated in a different way to phase A. Phase C is always longer than phase A, usually between 35 and 45 minutes. For our example let's say phase C is 6300 metres and you have 35 minutes to complete it and the speed is 180 metres/minute. As you have just finished your steeplechase phase, allow the horse to slow down gradually. If you allow 6 minutes for your first kilometre and 5 minutes for the rest, this will still bring you into the 10-minute box 2 minutes 30 seconds early, allowing you to walk for a longer period of time in phase C than you did in phase A. 180 metres/minute is slower than trotting speed but faster than walk. On phase C you will also have the 10-minute halt or C box. Depending on the weather conditions, the ground jury can decide that the 10-minute halt can be anything from zero to 10 minutes. It makes no difference what time you arrive in the 10-minute halt area, but once you are in there you have to stay for the allotted time until you can continue the rest of phase C. The time of the 10-minute halt is calculated into the time of phase C.

HOW DO YOU SAVE TIME ON A COURSE?

The fewer strides your horse takes as he goes around the cross country course, the quicker he will be. Obviously that doesn't mean taking out strides in a combination and it doesn't mean galloping flat out from one fence to another. What it does mean is walking the course properly and working out the most economical line to take around that course. If your horse has been trained correctly there will be no need to take wide sweeping turns into fences, as this will only add to your time. The shortest distance between two points is a straight line, and that is what you should try to achieve (Figure 2.3). I don't think of riding a course from one fence to another, I ride from one fence to the next point of rebalancing. The point at which you start rebalancing will depend on several factors: the horse and his level of training, the type of fence and the ground conditions. A simple ascending oxer fence will need less

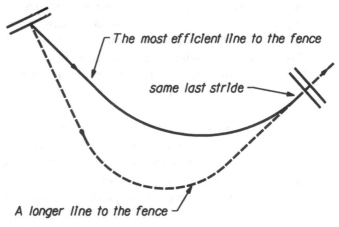

Figure 2.3   Two options for the route you can take to a fence are shown. Whichever route you choose, the final few strides will be the same.

rebalancing than an arrowhead complex, but I will always rebalance to some degree before each fence.

TROUBLESHOOTING

Q: How many times would you look at your watch at a novice ODE?
I probably only look at my watch three times on a one-day event course. Before I set off I will have a rough idea of where the half-way point is, so I will look at it then and possibly twice more on the latter half of the course.

Q: My horse is quite strong. Should I let him gallop on in the first half of the course in the hope he will be more settled on the second half?
No, absolutely not. Riding a cross country course is about riding each fence correctly and safely at the right speed. I don't allow a horse to gallop off because he wants to: if anything, the more he wants to gallop too fast the more I will say 'No'. I am the one who has walked the course so I know what it is like, and therefore it is my job to ride the horse at the correct pace all the way round the course. The other point is that with most horses, especially Thoroughbreds, allowing them to 'gallop fast' for a couple of minutes at the start of the course is not going to tire them out – it would take a lot more than that. All it would achieve would be a horse jumping fences in a fast, flat and very unsafe way.

Riding cross country safely and efficiently

RIDE SAFELY

To ride cross country safely your horse must be taught two very basic but very important things: go forward and come back. It's as simple as that. If they don't go forward at the precise moment you tell them to, the chances are they might not have the impulsion to get over some fences. If they don't come back to you in front of a fence there is a good chance the fence will be jumped flat and fast which could lead to a fall. This sort of control ties in with being able to adjust your take-off spot, by asking your horse to go on or come back to you. Once your horse has mastered these two basic skills you will be able to gallop on between fences knowing you can easily bring him back and rebalance in front of each fence.

RIDE EFFICIENTLY

To ride cross country efficiently you need to take the least number of strides over the whole course. Every stride will add to the time you take to complete the course. This doesn't mean you should take strides out of set distances in a combination – obviously it would be crazy to try to bounce a one-stride combination. It does mean you shouldn't make unnecessary wide sweeping loops as you ride the course. Learn to walk the course correctly and be clear about what speed you need to ride each fence. If fences eight to twelve, for example, require a fair amount of rebalancing you will probably fall behind your time, so you must know where you can make up that time elsewhere on the course. You must know where your point of rebalancing is before each fence so you don't start to slow down too early or too late. You must also be flexible in your plan of how you ride the course. If you have a problem at a fence it may influence the way you ride the rest of the course.

WHAT SPEED AM I TRAVELLING AT?

It is important to learn what speed you are travelling at. This is some-thing that should be learnt at home or at clinics, not at your first one-day event. The more eventing you do, the more you will acquire your per-sonal in-built clock. Until then the best way to learn what speed you are travelling at is to mark out a set area in a large paddock. Remember when you do this that you must have a flying start, and that doesn't mean coming out of an imaginary start box at a million miles an hour! Start cantering some distance before the start so that by the time you come past the marker you will be in your cross country canter. It will take some time to get a feel for the speed, and just when you have mastered that speed you will find yourself moving up the ladder where a slightly faster speed is required.

If it is possible include a jump in your speed training. It will help two-fold. It gives you the practice of rebalancing your horse whilst gallop-ing, and it also gives you an idea of the difference a jump will make to your overall speed. As you do this sort of training more often, you will start to get a feel for speed and the pace you are travelling at. Remember, however well your training goes at home, things will be different when you get to an event. Other factors have to be taken into account. Is it a hilly course? Or is it a twisty course? What are the ground conditions like? All these factors have to be considered when you walk the course, and then you must ride accordingly.

KEEP YOUR EYE ON THE FENCE

Keeping your eye on the fence as you ride towards it is, along with rebalancing, one of the most important things you can do. If you don't look at the fence, how can you expect to see a good stride to it? I don't advocate looking at a tree in the background, or a patch on the ground as you ride into a fence. I believe your eye has to be on the top rail of a vertical or the front rail of an oxer so that you can judge your distance to the fence. Start looking at the fence as early as possible, then keep look-ing at it all the way in, as it is harder to judge a good take-off spot if you look at the fence, look away and then look back.

The idea that you can look beyond the fence and leave the horse to decide the take-off spot is really unfair. You are the one who has walked the course, you know the distances between combinations, so it is your job to help the horse. He doesn't know that there's a drop after the ver-tical or a bounce after the palisade – you do. If you are told to look up at a tree to stop your body going too far forward as you ride over a fence you are really complicating the problem. If you are looking at the tree you will not be able to see a good take-off spot. I believe you must practice keeping your body in a good position so that your eyes can do what they need to do which is look at the fence.

If you are inclined to rush your horse into a fence and you look into the distance in an effort to avoid rushing, ask yourself why you are rushing. Is the fence difficult? Is your horse likely to stop and that's why you're going quickly? If this is the case, which it usually is, you might have to ride more aggressively into the fence, but you still need to look at it to have any chance of finding a good take-off spot. If you don't look at it, the chances are the horse could jump the fence badly and start to lose confidence, which will only escalate the problem.

REBALANCING

Rebalancing a horse, in the simplest terms, means slowing him down to bring him back to the required speed from which you will be able to jump each fence. When you start to walk the course with some knowledge, each fence will tell you what particular speed is required to jump it. The amount of rebalancing needed will depend on each individual fence. Rebalancing also puts the horse into a better shape, which will enable him to be more manoeuvrable for the rider, and he should go on to make a better, easier and safer jump over the fence. As well as the type of fence influencing the amount of rebalancing, each horse is different. For one horse rebalancing might simply require you, the rider, to sit up, and that alone will slow him down, whereas you may have to give several fairly strong half halts to a keen, strong horse before he changes his outline and speed.

Rebalancing the horse should only take three or four strides – any more than that and you are losing valuable time. Therefore, if it takes eight or nine strides to get your horse's outline and speed to the desired level, you need to do more training or look into using a stronger bit.

Training your horse to rebalance

Training your horse to rebalance on the cross country course is no different to flat work training carried out in the dressage arena; the only difference is the speed at which you are travelling. Because of this you must be strict with yourself and your horse. It's no good allowing the horse to take an extra few strides to rebalance because by then you could have arrived at the fence and it would be too late. If you have had to start rebalancing a long way out from the fence you're just wasting time.

Once your horse's training has reached the level where you can increase and decrease his canter in the arena, you are ready to move up a gear and practise in an open paddock. When you are in your cross country position ask your horse to increase his canter speed by softening the contact and encouraging him forward with your leg and, if necessary, your spurs. Allow him to gallop, in a good rhythm, for a short distance and then bring him back to you by sitting up, and using half halts. I find it easier to rebalance my horse in a light seat and I then keep this position all the way into the fence. You may have to use a deeper seat if your horse is a little stronger. When you have rebalanced your horse, use your leg and hand to keep him at the desired speed. After you have travelled at this speed for a short distance ask him to gallop on again before once again rebalancing. This simple exercise should help you to approach your cross country fences in a way that is safe for both you and your horse.

If no attempt is made to rebalance on the cross country course, you will be more likely to arrive at the fence too fast, too flat or both, and the horse will be paying little attention to the fence in front of him. Once you have jumped a fence it's fine to gallop on as long as you know where your next point of rebalancing is before the next fence, and provided the horse does not spot the next jump and either run or

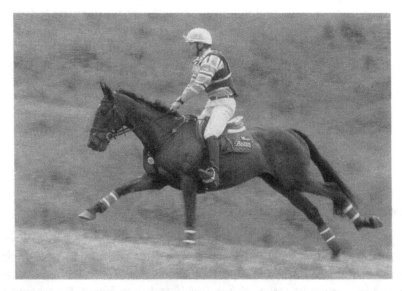

Figure 3.1 This photograph shows just how long a horse's stride can be, which is why it's important to rebalance and shorten your horse's canter so it will be easier to find a good take-off spot and jump a fence safely.

stall to it. It is important to realise that you should be galloping to your next point of rebalance, not to the next fence. If you gallop straight to the next fence you won't have allowed any space to rebalance, so make sure when you walk the course that you know where your points of rebalancing are before each fence. At times, the fence and the point of rebalancing will be on the same line.

Rebalancing downhill

To illustrate my training I rode two very different horses: one very green, Caro, the other experienced, Ava.

Caro

Caro is a 6 year old, three-quarters Warmblood, one-quarter Thoroughbred mare, with a good trainable temperament. Before having her foal, which had been weaned from her about 4 months before the photographs were taken, she had been broken in but had not competed at all. A few weeks before this photo shoot, Caro had taken part in her first event which was at pre-novice level, so a true to life cross country training session is illustrated.

Ava

Ava is a 9 year old half Warmblood, half Thoroughbred mare who was in preparation for the Jerez World Equestrian Games. She has competed successfully at three and four star level, so she is very experienced. Because I wasn't planning to take Ava to an event before departing overseas, this cross country training was part of her preparation. She is a snaffled mouth, very soft, easy horse to ride cross country, with a great focus and brain.

If I am confident that my horse will listen to my rebalancing (or slowing down) aids, I would generally rebalance about six strides out from the fence, once again depending on the difficulty of the fence. Galloping downhill could make rebalancing harder, and it may take you longer, as horses tend to be running on a little more, often going onto the forehand. Because of this, when approaching a fence on a downhill, I generally allow a little longer to rebalance.

In Figures 3.2–3.5 you can see Caro galloping downhill. When I ask her to slow down she puts in an objection. This can be seen by the way she twists her head (Figure 3.3) and then puts her head in the air (Figure 3.4). However, a few strides later (Figure 3.5) she has settled down, slowed

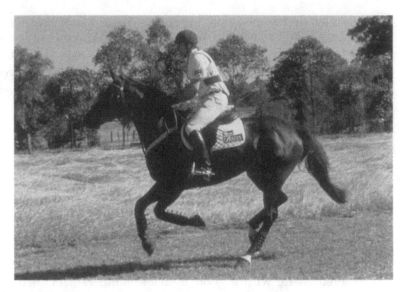

Figure 3.2

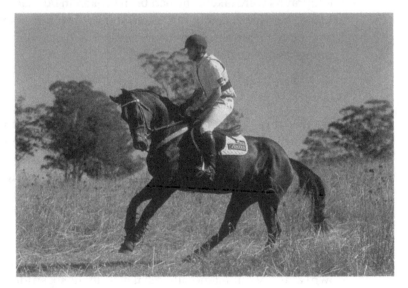

Figure 3.3

down and is now quite happy to go on at the new speed. Note how her whole outline is more together in Figure 3.5 than in Figure 3.2 where she is quite open. I might have to go through the objection in the middle photos for four or five strides until the horse understands what I am asking her to do and she is able to do it. The first time I asked Caro to rebalance on the downhill it took me around seven strides to get back to

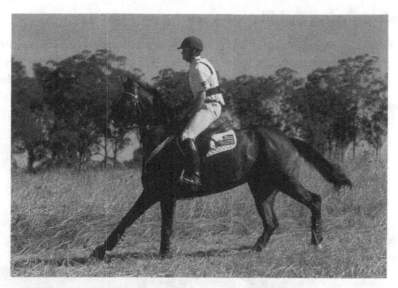

Figure 3.4

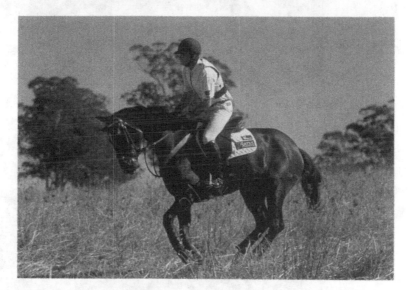

Figure 3.5

the pace I wanted. After repeating the exercise a few times, she rebalanced in three strides. As the horse starts to understand and be less surprised by the exercise, the resistance to rebalancing will be reduced. Obviously, as Caro competes more she will become better at rebalancing. You must practise what you want your horse to do. You can't just expect him to listen to you on the first half halt if he has not been trained to do so.

Rebalancing uphill

Rebalancing when travelling uphill is usually a little easier as the horse is more likely to be travelling in a better shape with less weight on his front end. Figures 3.6–3.9 show how open Caro's stride was before I rebalanced and how after rebalancing she looks in a good outline to be

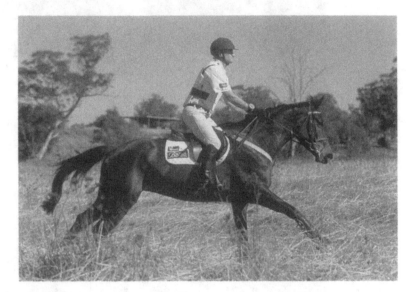

Figure 3.6

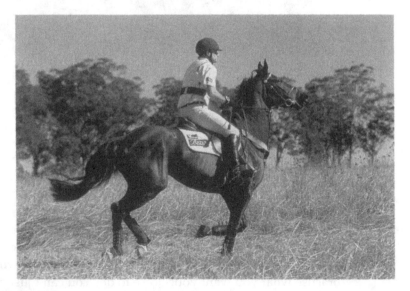

Figure 3.7

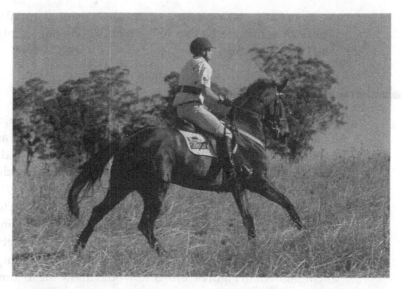

Figure 3.8

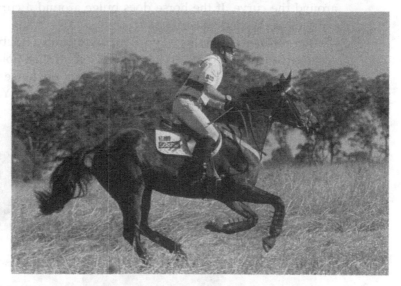

Figure 3.9

approaching a fence. At novice level or above, you could expect to find a fence either half way up a hill or on top of the hill. Regardless of the type of fence, it is important to rebalance your horse on the hill so he is able to jump the fence without struggling. If you gallop up the hill and into the fence without rebalancing, it is quite possible the horse will either jump the fence flatly, risking injury, or simply run out of impulsion and stop. It must be remembered that uphill fences are taller simply because the take-off spot is lower.

Rebalancing on a curve

When you are jumping a fence with a curving approach, use the curve to your advantage by rebalancing on the curve. As well as slowing the horse down, it will allow you to look at the fence and get the best possible line to it. It is important to know when to start riding the curve, which may also be the rebalancing point.

In Figures 3.10–3.12 you can see that Caro has listened to my rebalancing aids to slow down and is now quite happily travelling on towards the fence. I must continue to stress that the amount of rebalancing I do will depend on the type of fence I am jumping. For example, the rebalancing shown in Figures 3.10–3.12 would allow me to jump a fence in a very controlled way. To ride the curve I used my outside aids, both leg and hand, to stop any bulging, which could happen when you ride around the curve. If the horse does bulge around a curve it is much harder to see a good take-off point.

After rebalancing in this way I went on to jump a double of logs at a distance of 13.1 metres (43 ft) in three very controlled holding strides. I would choose to ride a combination like this if my horse was inexperienced or I wanted to keep her very much under control. You can see the

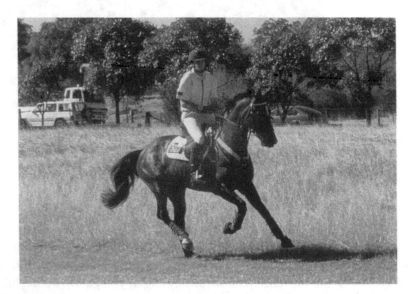

Figure 3.10

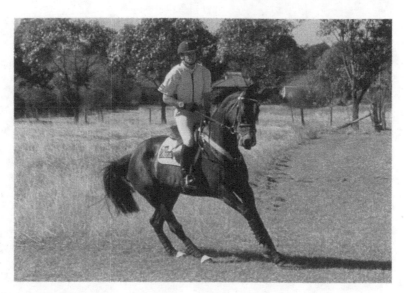

Figure 3.11

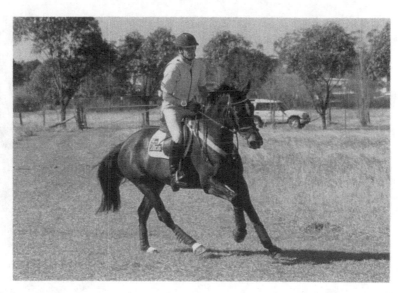

Figure 3.12

jump over the first log was very neat (Figure 3.13) and that I'm going to land quite close to the back of the first fence which will allow me to fit in three holding strides between the logs. If, on the other hand, the horse was more experienced, I trusted her not to try and run out of the side of the fence, or I was trying to make up some time, I would choose to ride

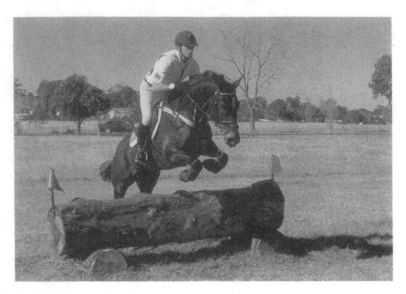

Figure 3.13

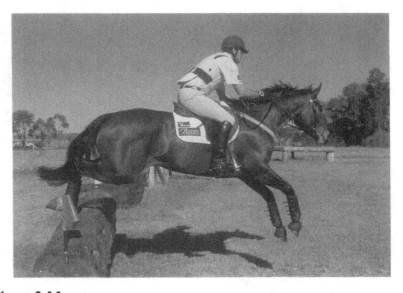

Figure 3.14

the combination on a forward two strides (Figure 3.14). Riding this way, I would not need to rebalance to the same extent as in the previous option. The horse would jump the fence bigger, landing further out as shown in Figure 3.14 which would bring me closer to the next fence so that I could easily ride the combination in two strides.

Some rebalancing should take place before every fence. Don't think you can gallop round a corner and jump a fence without making any effort to rebalance your horse. You may get away with it over logs at a small height, but it will not help the horse's confidence and may lead to an accident as you move up the grades. When you are riding a curve to a more difficult fence, the horse will need more time to access the fence, so you will need an approach which is straighter for longer.

If you want to save time . . .

The best way to save time is to take the least number of strides as you travel around the course. That doesn't mean riding a two-stride double in one gigantic stride because you are likely to fall, but it does mean reading the course and walking the most economical route. I don't jump a fence and gallop on aiming for the next fence. I jump a fence and gallop on aiming for my next point of rebalancing before the next fence. I will decide where that point of rebalancing shall be when I walk the course.

TYPES OF FENCES

Every fence you see on a cross country course can be related to a certain basic type of fence. For example, the magnificent aboriginal snake fence at the Sydney Olympics looked amazing, but at the end of the day it was just a palisade over a ditch, so if your horse is confident over a ditch and palisade the fact that the fence looks so bright and colourful shouldn't make any difference. Most cross country fences will fit into one of the following categories.

Ascending oxers

These fences are lower in front than behind, making them one of the easiest to jump because they follow the same shape that a horse would naturally make over a fence. Ascending oxers also allow the horse's front legs to work more slowly. It is important to look at the front rail as you approach the fence, even though it is slightly lower. Types of fences in this category could include logs, if large, and table fences.

Square oxers

These fences are the same height in front and behind, making them a little harder to jump because the horse has to pick up his front legs very quickly and neatly in time to clear the front rail. Square oxers could include parallel rails.

Uprights or verticals

Uprights are generally more difficult for a horse to jump because they allow less room for error in the way a horse assesses his own height effort and how he picks up his front legs. The higher and more vertical the fence, the slower and more controlled your approach should be. The more ground line there is, the easier the fence will be to jump, as the ground line will give a better view of the fence. When a horse jumps a spread like an oxer, he jumps the front rail and the back rail, and his natural arc will take him above the height of the fence. However, when a horse jumps a vertical, the fence doesn't influence the height he makes with his body at all. Because of this you must take more time approaching a vertical to give yourself a better chance of getting a good take-off spot. Some verticals have sloping faces, like a steeplechase fence, which make them easier to jump than a normal upright. Although a large log fence is usually thought of as an ascending oxer, if the log was smaller in diameter and suspended in the air it could come into the category of a vertical fence.

Triple bars

Some triple bars, depending on their slope, could also be classed as ascending oxers with an extra rail in the middle (Figure 3.15). A classic triple bar has three rails which, when looked at from the side, are approximately at a forty five degree angle to the ground. Another fence which could fall into two categories is a steeplechase fence, which could be called a sloping vertical (Figure 3.15) or a triple bar.

Triple Bars

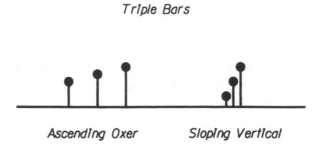

Ascending Oxer   *Sloping Vertical*

Figure 3.15 A triple bar can be classed as an ascending oxer with an extra rail in the middle, or a sloping vertical such as a steeplechase fence.

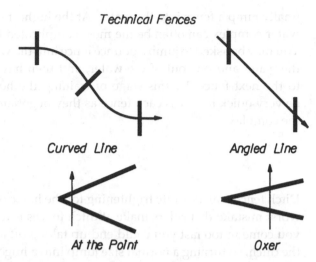

Figure 3.16   Accuracy is very important when you are jumping technical fences such as the ones shown here.

Accuracy or technical fences

Arrowheads and apexes are both accuracy questions. Arrowheads have a very narrow facing front, giving the horse ample opportunity to run off the fence to either side. Of course, if they have a wing on one side they are less likely to run out to that side. Apexes or corners can cause horses to run off the pointed end of the fence. They are both accuracy questions because the rider and the horse must be able to keep a very good line into each fence, jumping it in exactly the right place. Technical fences can also include fences like offset brushes or rails which have to be jumped on an angle with the rider again required to keep a good line, or fences on curves (Figure 3.16).

Steps up and down

Steps or banks up and down can feature on a cross country course as a single fence or multiple fences, for example, three steps up or down. Steps up or down can also be part of a combination fence.

Water

At lower grades, the water fence may require you to simply walk down a slope into water and jump out or even slope out. Gradually as you move up the grades you will be asked to drop into the water, and finally jump a fence into the water. At the highest level of eventing the water complex can often be the most complicated fence on the course. You may be asked to jump a bounce fence into the water, jump a fence in the water and one out of the water, and then have a related distance to the next fence. By this stage of training the horse and rider must be very quick to assess each fence as they negotiate their way through the complex.

Ditches

Ditch fences can be quite frightening for the horse or rider, or both. The worst mistake that riders make at ditch fences is to come in too fast. If you come in too fast you could end up taking off a long way out from the ditch, so turning a normal size jump into a huge effort. Ditch fences can range from an open ditch to a ditch and rail, ditch and brush or palisade, or a ditch as part of a combination. A ditch palisade is simply a vertical with a good ground line. To get a good take-off spot if you are riding an open ditch, look at the front rail or ground line of the ditch. If you are riding an oxer over a ditch, look at the front rail.

Combinations

All the various fences you and your horse will be asked to jump on the cross country course will be one of the above fences or a combination of several of them. For example, you may come across a bank up, followed a stride later by an upright brush, followed by a drop down to an arrowhead. This is where walking the course is vital, as it is at this time you will decide how to approach each fence. Regardless of what type of fence you are approaching you will have to do some sort of organising and rebalancing.

Bear in mind that the horse's normal stride length is 3.6 metres (12 ft). This stride length may need to be varied, as necessary, from 3 metres (10 ft) to 3.96 metres (13 ft) when jumping certain combinations. The striding in combinations will be determined by the distance between them, the type of fence, both in and out, and the ground conditions. The jump itself dictates the speed at which it should be ridden. If the fence is a combination, it will further depend on the distance of that combination. In other words, a short bounce distance will be ridden with slightly less speed than a long bounce. A triple bar or ascending oxer will need a different approach to an apex or arrowhead. Regardless of what standard of horse I am riding or the speed I am travelling cross country, I will rebalance and reorganise before every fence, and aim to jump each fence efficiently and effectively.

Rebalancing and keeping your eye on the fence are two of the most important things you have to do on a cross country course. Rebalancing will put your horse into a better shape and speed from which he will be able to jump the fence. Keeping your eye on the fence will give you the best chance of choosing a good take-off spot. If you rebalance and keep your eye on the fence you will be well on the way to achieving a safe cross country round.

GETTING STARTED

The start

Before you get to the start box, you should allow a short time to warm up your horse. Start off by walking your horse for a few minutes before working him in trot and canter on both reins. As you do this make sure your horse is listening to you and is happy to speed up, slow down, turn right and left. I know it all sounds simple, but really that is all you have to do when you are riding cross country. If your horse starts to get a little keen, ride several transitions to get his brain back to thinking along the correct lines. If your horse doesn't naturally want to gallop, give him a short gallop in the warm-up area to get him thinking forward. Sometimes the size of the warm-up area might restrict this, but you should have enough space for a short burst. Depending on your horse, you might decide to trot over the practice fence the first time before coming in at a canter. Once you have jumped the fence a couple of times, ask the horse to come in with a shorter more balanced canter and then a stronger more forward canter, always making sure you are in control before and after the fence. By the time you are called into the start box your horse should be warmed up and listening to you.

If you are planning on completing the cross country course within the time allowed, it is essential to have a good start. All horses are different, but most of them, once they have been round a few cross country courses, know what is coming as they stand in the start box and they tend to get a bit uptight. Try to avoid this, if possible, by keeping your horse walking until you can walk into the start box and set off. If the horse sets off out of the start box like a raging bull, you might come to grief at the first combination fence where the horse isn't yet settled. If your horse is settled you will be able to start out of the start box and quickly build up to a good speed, which is relevant to the level at which you are competing. However, if the first fence is quite close to the start you should set off at a steadier speed and be prepared to make up the time elsewhere on the course. Young or inexperienced horses have to be taught about cross country, so again the speed might be a little slower depending on the circumstances. There are some horses who are quite content to canter around the course and have to be taught to gallop, and occasionally some of this teaching has to be done on the cross country course itself.

A good course designer will try to give you a confident start on the course by making the first few fences fairly straightforward. This should be the case whether it is an advanced track or an introductory course. A straightforward fence is one which does not require a great deal of rebalancing, that is providing the horse is travelling across the ground in a fairly balanced way. Most straightforward fences are ascending oxers or sloping verticals of one sort or another, for example, this could be a log, a steeplechase type fence, or perhaps ascending rails.

A log fence, as shown in Figure 3.17, is often used as a first fence, and it won't matter too much if you get a good spot or get in a little deep at this type of fence as it is fairly forgiving and the horse should jump it easily. After jumping a few straightforward fences at the start of the course, where you have rebalanced to a lesser degree, you may find your horse doesn't immediately respond to you when you ask him to rebalance more seriously before the first complex fence. This is something you must be aware of, so be sure to allow plenty of time for him to rebalance and try to have him travelling the way you want before you get to the fence.

As you go around the course

It is essential for the horse to use his brain as he goes around the course, as this will give him the best possible chance of negotiating each obstacle successfully, so the rider must concentrate on the job in hand for the whole length of the course. You must also try to be aware of what your horse may be thinking. If you have a problem at one fence, how will the horse react to the next fence? Will he be feeling less confident and think of stopping? Or did he get a fright and will he try to rush the next fence? All these questions and answers will become easier to you the more you get to know your horse.

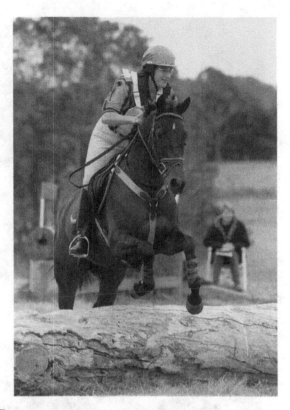

Figure 3.17

JUMPING A SLOPING VERTICAL FENCE

As I said previously, this type of fence is one of the most forgiving, as it will allow the horse to jump the fence whether he takes off from a normal take-off spot, or one that is too close, or a far away spot – provided the fence is not too wide. Because the fence is lower in front than behind, it follows the natural shape the horse makes over a jump. Even if he doesn't lift his front legs up very neatly, it will not usually cause a problem because the shape of the fence will allow him more time to get his legs out of the way.

In Figure 3.18 Caro is coming into a steeplechase fence on a long stride. Consequently she takes off to jump the fence from quite a long way out (Figure 3.19) and makes a flatter but acceptable shape over the fence (Figure 3.20). She will also be landing further out from the back of the fence because of the speed of approach and the flatter jump. Although it isn't too much of a problem to take off too far away from

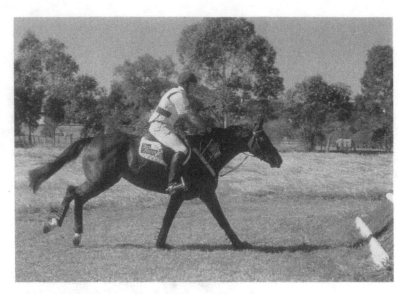

Figure 3.18

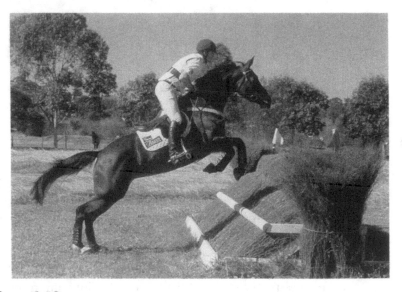

Figure 3.19

this type of fence, you must learn to choose your take-off spot for a reason, and not just use the same take-off spot for all types of fences. In your training, practise riding at different speeds and be able to choose different take-off spots because this will enable you to be able to jump each fence more efficiently.

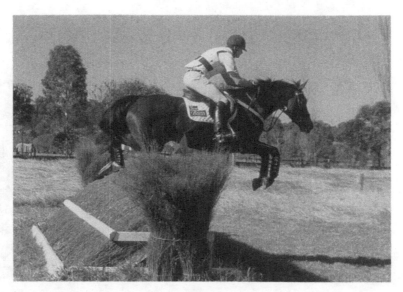

Figure 3.20

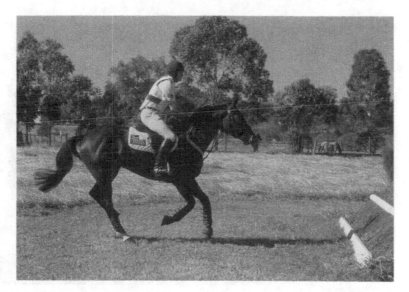

Figure 3.21

Now we see the fence jumped again, but this time I have rebalanced the horse more so the canter is a little shorter (Figure 3.21) and I am able to ride closer to the bottom of the fence for a deep take-off spot (Figure 3.22). This type of fence allows longer for the front legs to get up, which they are by the time she is at the top of the fence. Notice the

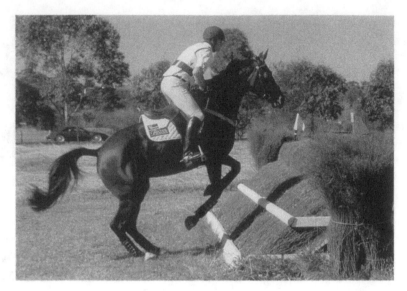

Figure 3.22

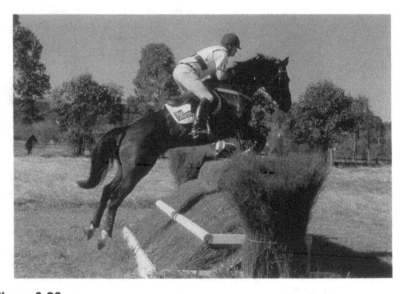

Figure 3.23

difference in the shape the horse makes between the deeper take-off spot and the further away spot in the previous photos. Because the horse got closer to the fence in Figure 3.23 she has jumped up in the air more, as opposed to the flat style in Figure 3.20.

Explanation: The take-off spot is the point at which the horse leaves the ground to jump the fence. A deep spot is when you take off close to the fence. An away spot is when you take off further away from the fence.

JUMPING TECHNICAL FENCES LIKE ANGLED BRUSHES

As you ride around the course you have several choices of how you could jump each fence, although hopefully all these decisions will have been made during your course walk. The way you rebalance and ride into each fence will determine how the fence is jumped. The fence I'm tackling next is an offset or angled brush fence with a very short two strides in between the first and second elements. Figure 3.24 shows the angle of the fence from the air.

The faster approach

In this sequence of photos I have come into the first brush with a little speed and have kept some feel of the horse's mouth over the fence (Figure 3.25) encouraging Caro to land shorter, which she does. I then keep a feel of her mouth all the way through the combination (Figure 3.26) until we take off for the second element. Because I have come in with some speed, Caro takes off for the second fence from quite a deep spot and her front legs are coming up late (Figure 3.27), but because I am decreasing speed at this stage she has time to get them out of the way. She goes on to make a nice but slightly flat jump over the second element (Figure 3.28). If you want to jump a combination on a holding stride, it is important that the first landing stride is short to allow the horse room to put in the required strides as you decrease

The Angled Brushes

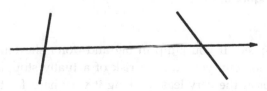

Figure 3.24 The position of the angled brushes from the air.

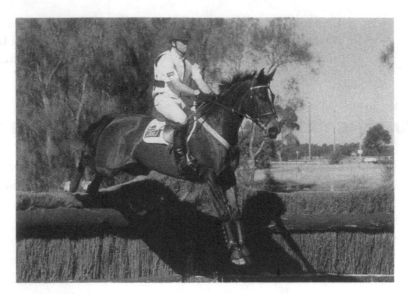

Figure 3.25

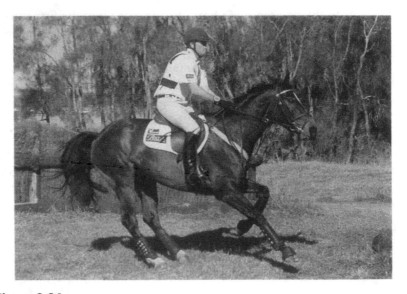

Figure 3.26

speed. If you jump in big and don't shorten the stride until the last moment, you run the risk of actually stopping the horse altogether, or at the very least making it very hard for the horse to get over the second fence.

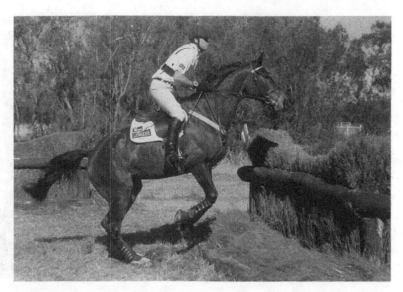

Figure 3.27

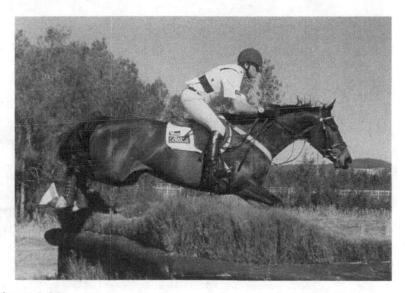

Figure 3.28

The slower approach

In the second sequence I have rebalanced much more than I did for the previous approach and allowed Caro more freedom over the fence (Figure 3.29), which allows her to jump well out over the first element (Figure 3.30). I then ride softly between the fences (Figures 3.31, 3.32),

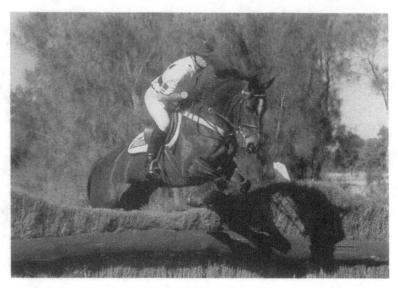

Figure 3.29

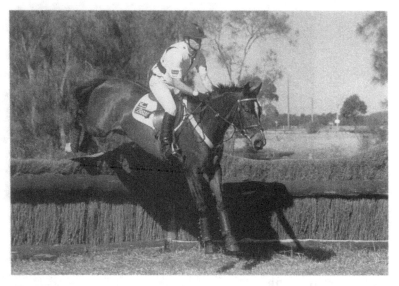

Figure 3.30

keeping her balanced, and she gets a good take-off spot which is a little close to the ground line but good for a vertical, and goes onto make a good shape (Figure 3.33) and jump over the second element (Figure 3.34). If you rebalance and slow down before the first fence of a combination it will mean less work for you and your horse in between each fence.

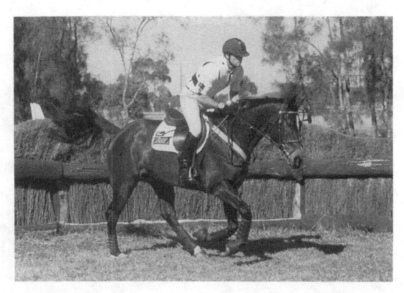

Figure 3.31

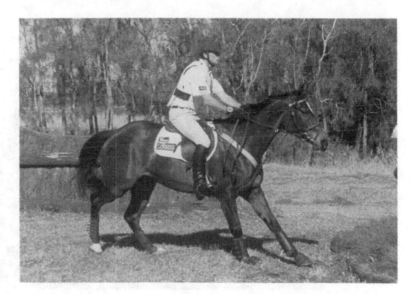

Figure 3.32

The importance of a good lower leg position
A good lower leg position will make you much more secure as a rider
when you jump over fences. I don't opt for an exaggerated forward
lower leg position, but regardless of what the top half of my body is
doing (leaning backwards or forwards) I do try to keep my weight

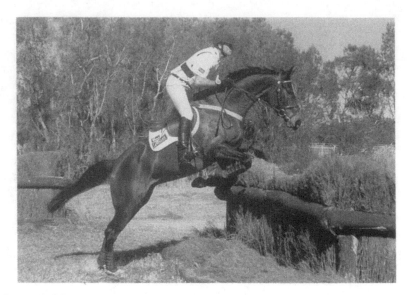

Figure 3.33

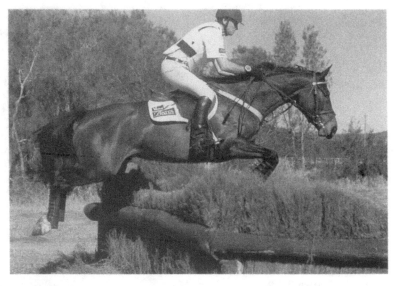

Figure 3.34

down through my lower legs so my position is secure. Riders who let their heels come up and start balancing on their knees will have trouble remaining in place should the horse have a problem, such as pecking on landing.

STEPS UP OR DOWN

If the steps or banks are vertical, you can treat them just as you would any other vertical or upright fence, the only difference being that the horse lands half way through the jump. If the bank has a good ground line it will jump more like a vertical with a ground line which again ends half way through. The worst mistake you can make is to complicate fences too much. Break them down into what type of fence they actually are and then ride them appropriately.

Most horses jump up and down banks quite happily, but some are inclined to scramble up a bank and land in a bit of a heap. If you find your horse is slightly unsure about jumping up and down banks, find a small safe bank and simply practise going up and down, making sure that you stay in balance. If the bank is small, there is no need to throw yourself into an exaggerated forward seat going uphill and an exaggerated backward seat going downhill.

Caro jumps up the bank in quite a nice way for a green horse (Figure 3.35) and I keep the contact whilst allowing her enough freedom to balance herself when she lands on top (Figure 3.36). As we jump down the bank I stay in a balanced position and because it is a small bank I don't find it necessary to slip my reins (Figure 3.37). By doing this I am able to keep the canter when we land without having to make too many alterations to my position.

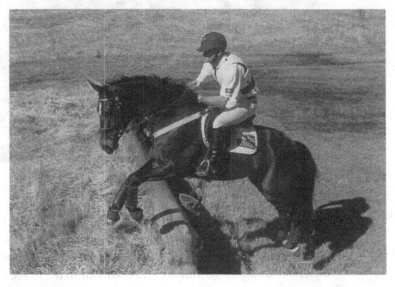

Figure 3.35

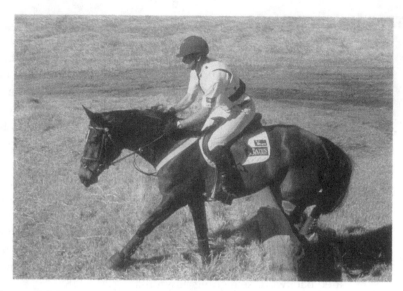

Figure 3.36

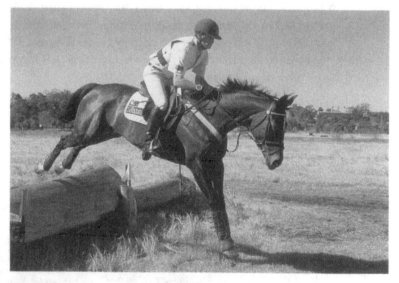

Figure 3.37

When you start off jumping up and down banks try to stay sitting quietly in your usual jumping position and after a few sessions the horse should have worked out what to do with his legs, without too much fuss. Don't move onto a bigger bank until the horse is happy at the lower level.

BULLFINCH

A bullfinch has whispy brush in the top of the fence which you can brush through. For example, the solid part of the fence might be a metre high, but with the added thin brush it could be 1.20 metres. Although the rider knows his horse can brush though the top of the fence, some horses don't realise this and inexperienced horses will often try to jump the full height of the fence, 1.20 metres. Therefore be prepared for a big jump if you are on an inexperienced or careful horse. After horses have jumped a few bullfinches they usually get the idea that they don't have to jump the full height, but some will always be a bit careful. It is important if you are riding a green horse or a careful horse that you come into a bullfinch with a strong enough canter to jump 1.20 metres if you think he will want to jump the lot.

In Figure 3.38 you can see Caro showing her inexperience as she jumps well above the necessary height, only brushing through the fence slightly. As long as you have approached in the right canter this is not a real problem. At the other extreme, in Figure 3.39 you can see a much more experienced horse who is quite happy to jump through the thinner brush.

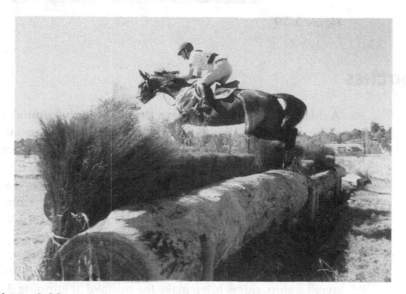

Figure 3.38

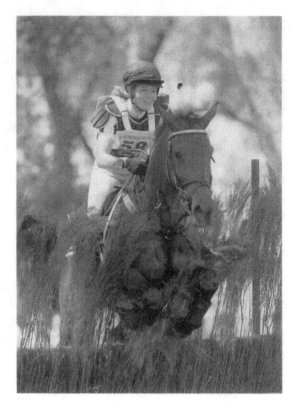

Figure 3.39

DITCHES

A ditch can be anything from a large hole in the ground, to a ditch and rail, a ditch and palisade, or a ditch and brush. It is crucial when you are jumping a large fence to get a good take-off spot. For example, if you are jumping a wide ditch and you take off 0.61 metres (2 ft) away from the front of the ditch it makes it a 0.6 metre bigger ditch; if the ditch is 1.8 metres (6 ft) wide and you take off 0.6 metres away from it, it becomes a 2.4 metre (8 ft) ditch, and to that end if you take off 1.8 metres before the ditch you will end up jumping a very big fence!

Ditch fences can often be big and imposing, and many riders worry about their horses spooking at the hole in the ground. In an attempt to avoid a stop, riders often make the mistake of jumping ditch fences too fast in the hope that the horse will have no option but to jump the fence. This has at least one big disadvantage. In the majority of cases as the horse goes faster his stride gets longer, which allows the rider fewer options for a good take-off spot. He will either take off a long way out, or chip in a very short stride, or shuffle in front of the fence or, of course, he could be lucky and get it just right, but it's all a bit disorganised. You don't need speed if the ditch is very wide, you just need a balanced canter that gives you the option to move up a little in the last couple of strides after you have seen the take-off spot. If you are already travelling fast you may not be able to move up closer if you have an away take-off spot.

Start training over small ditches so that you know you don't have to gallop at them and gradually build up to bigger ditches as the horse becomes more confident. I like to come into a ditch, having rebalanced and then be travelling in a good canter, that is a canter which gives me more options to choose a better take-off spot. The type of canter I have will also depend on the other fence, if there is one, which is behind the ditch. For example, if I'm jumping a ditch and palisade, I would need a good enough canter to be able to jump the palisade correctly. This type of fence is just a vertical with the ditch giving the fence a very good ground line.

A good take-off spot
You will know when you have jumped a fence from a good take-off spot because it will feel good, just as when you choose a bad one it will feel bad. A good take-off spot is a feeling, but you can't get that feeling if you don't look at the fence. A good take-off spot is also related to your canter. If you don't have a good canter you will find it much harder to see a good take-off spot. For example, if you are cantering to a fence in a long fast flat frame, you might actually see a good stride but it will be much harder to adjust a long canter stride than it would be to adjust a rebalanced better quality canter stride.

WATER

A water fence can be made up of various elements, and each part should be jumped accordingly. At lower levels, horses may be asked to simply walk into the water, turn around a flag and come out, but by pre-novice level and above you will usually have to jump a fence into the water. Many course designers use logs or roll tops as the fence into water because, being ascending oxers, they are more forgiving than uprights and allow more time for the horse's legs to come up.

You cannot hope to train over all the various types of fences which you will find on a cross country course, but two of the hardest obstacles

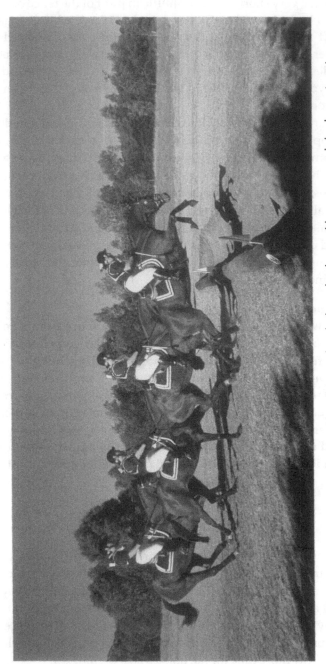

Figure 3.40 A very simple ditch being jumped by a young rider. The horse has been ridden quite strongly but been given time to see the ditch and goes on to jump it quite open, but well enough.

on the course tend to be the water and/or a ditch type fence. These fences should definitely be practised before an event so that both you and your horse build up some confidence without the added pressure of an actual competition. Puddle training is helpful and, although initially the horse might try everything possible to go around the puddle, perseverance and patience will usually work in the end. You must be sure that the footing in the water is very good, so there is no chance that the horse will slip. Make sure you ask the horse to enter the water in a sensible place and have thought your actions through. He must enter the water where you want, not where he wants. Once the horse is walking confidently through the water you can build up to a small jump in and out.

It is important to teach the horse to walk and then jump into and out of the water exactly where you want him to. Although this may not seem too vital early on in the horse's training, it will make all the difference as the horse moves up the grades where you may have to jump a log into the water, another fence in the water and possibly an arrowhead when you come out of the water. If you have allowed the horse to wander off the line you wanted to take, you run the risk of running out at one of the fences in the water complex, so be strict with yourself and your horse from day one.

Jumping a small drop into water should be no different to jumping a small drop without water, although the look of the water may spook some horses for the first few times. To build up the horse's confidence make sure he is happily walking in and out of water before you ask him to drop in, and always make sure the water you jump into is quite shallow with a good firm base. Landing in muddy holding ground can panic a horse, and he might not be easily persuaded to go into water the next time. The more horses jump into water, the more confident they will become and their style will improve.

You can see in Figure 3.41 how the inexperienced Caro has more or less stepped over the fence and is having a good look at the water. In Figure 3.42, Ava, the more experienced horse, has made a much better shape over the same fence, jumping confidently into the water.

In Figures 3.43 and 3.44, I have asked the horses to jump again into the water, this time over a roll top fence. Once again Caro shows her inexperience by crouching down on her hocks, having a good look at the water and not picking up her front legs very neatly. In comparison, Ava is looking much more confident with pricked ears as she jumps boldly into the water looking for the next fence which is a bank out.

The other thing Figures 3.41–3.44 show is the importance of a strong lower leg position. I don't tend to exaggerate my lower leg position, in other words I don't let my lower leg go too far forward, but I do keep the

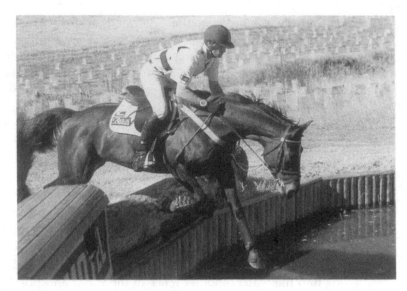

Figure 3.41

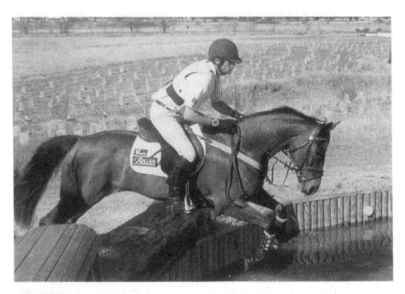

Figure 3.42

weight down through my legs which makes my position quite safe. If you let your lower legs move backwards over a fence they will automatically put the top half of your body further forward than necessary, and if the horse should hit a fence or peck on landing you are likely to be thrown forward.

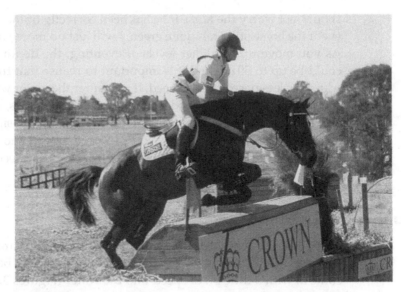

Figure 3.43

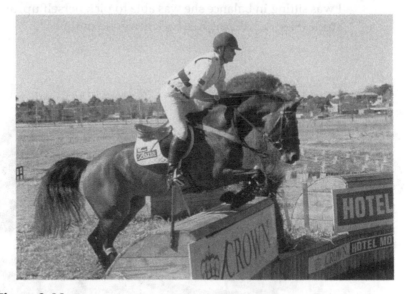

Figure 3.44

Does the water make a difference?

I ride a fence into water the same way I would as if it was not related to water. For example, if there was a 1.1 metre log dropping into water, I would ride it as a 1.1 metre log with a drop on the other side. The water should not worry the horse if he has been correctly trained, and if at an event the horse still feels quite green, I will just do more water training. As you move up to higher levels of eventing, the depth of the water could be up to 50 cm and it is important to realise that the deeper the water the less pace you will need. If you enter the water with too much speed there will be a tremendous drag on the horse's legs, he will not be able to move them as quickly as he would normally, possibly losing his balance and falling. Obviously, you will need a good enough canter to jump the fence into the water, but you certainly don't need to be going too fast into deep water.

Balance and position

In the next sequence of photos you can see how important it is to keep your balance during all the different stages of the jump. Because I have come in with a little bit of speed into the water (Figures 3.45, 3.46) and Caro is inexperienced she has landed a bit steep (Figure 3.47) and almost looks as if she is going to nose-dive into the water (Figure 3.48). Because I was sitting in balance she was able to pick herself up, and by the next stride (Figure 3.49) she was back in a good outline.

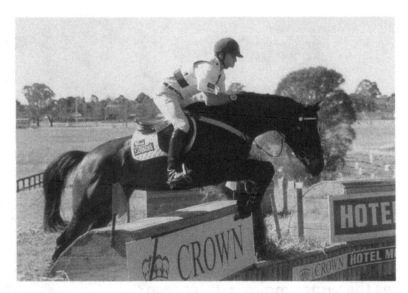

Figure 3.45

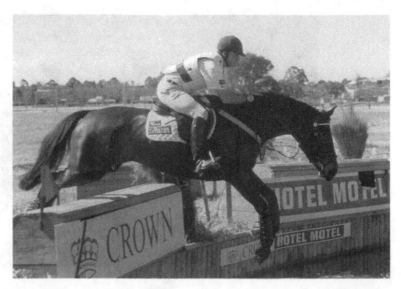

Figure 3.46

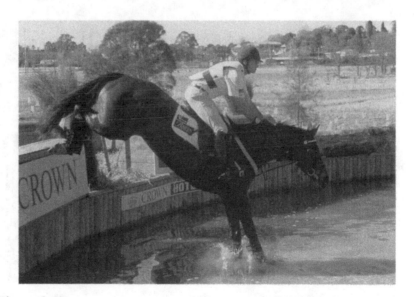

Figure 3.47

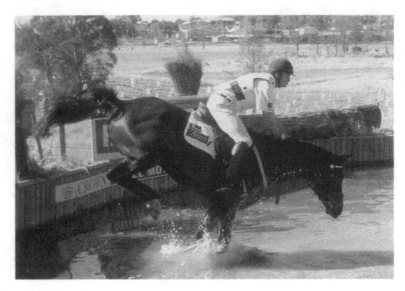

Figure 3.48

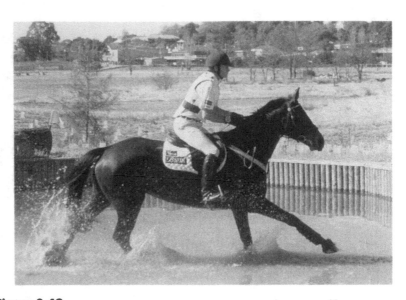

Figure 3.49

When I'm jumping a drop into water I don't find it necessary to adopt an exaggerated leaning back position, like the rider in Figure 3.50, unless the drop is very big. That's not to say it is a bad thing to lean back a little as you come into an ordinary drop fence into water, but it does mean that if you have something technical to ride in the water you

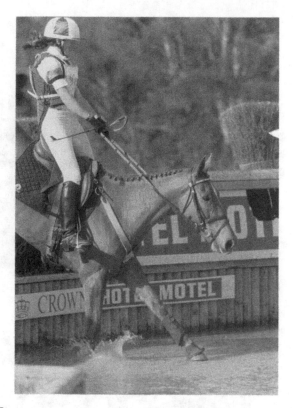

Figure 3.50

might not be in the best position to ride it, as you may have slipped your reins as you leant back and not have time to gather them back up. Whether that matters or not depends very much on the horse you are riding. Confident experienced horses will line up the next fence all by themselves, despite the rider not being able to give clear instructions, whereas some horses find long reins the perfect excuse to duck out of the side of the next fence.

In Figure 3.51 I have jumped into the water in an upright balanced position and would feel quite confident to tackle another fence straight away. In Figure 3.52 you can see that I am leaning back and have slipped the reins slightly, but certainly not as much as many riders would choose to do. Because of the still relatively short length of rein, I should be able to make a good approach to the next fence. Being able to adopt various positions is made easier when you ride in a flat seated saddle, whereas a saddle with a high cantle would influence my position too much.

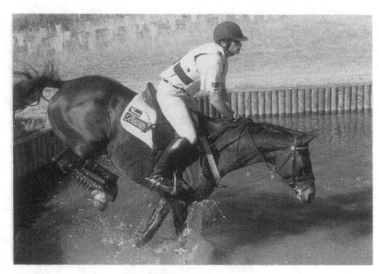

Figure 3.51

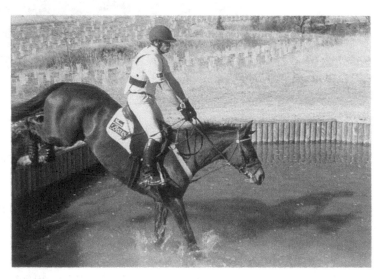

Figure 3.52

Getting out of the water

The step or bank out of water is again something that the inexperienced horse will need to practise. With the splash of the water some horses find it difficult to focus on the step and can end up clambering out, one leg at a time.

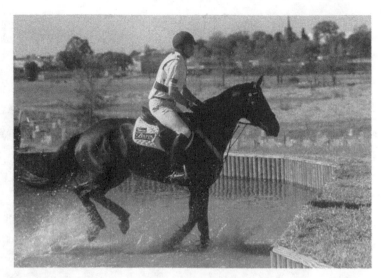

Figure 3.53

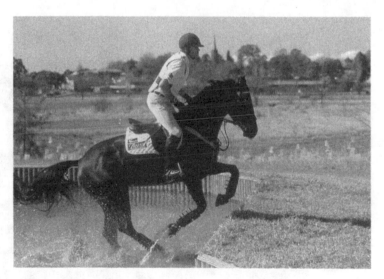

Figure 3.54

You can see in Figures 3.53 and 3.54 that as Caro comes through the water she is unsure of what to do next. When she comes up the bank out of the water her ears are back as she works out what she has to do with her legs. This clearly shows that an inexperienced horse wouldn't cope with another related fence after coming out of the water as it would be just too much for them to think about.

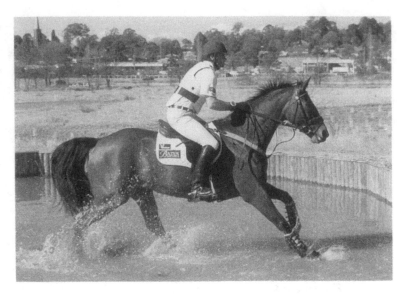

Figure 3.55

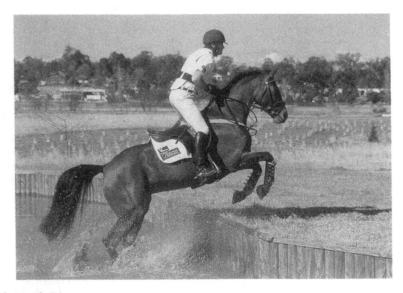

Figure 3.56

Compare Caro's photos with those of the experienced Ava who jumps up the bank neatly (Figure 3.55) and looks very focused (Figure 3.56) on what is coming up next, which was an arrowhead just beyond this photo frame.

TECHNICAL QUESTIONS – APEXES

As you move up to a higher level of eventing, the fences you will be asked to jump on the cross country course will become not only bigger but also more technical. A common technical fence is an apex or corner. These can be jumped as a single fence or on a related line to another fence. Looking at the shape of an apex, it is obvious that the main problem in jumping this type of fence is the high risk of a run-out to the pointed end if you don't choose a good line.

You have two choices when jumping these apexes (Figure 3.57). You can either jump the fence square to the fence with the horse's body straight, the advantage of this choice being that you are less likely to run out as you will be jumping a fence which appears to the horse to be an ordinary oxer. The disadvantage is the extra time it will take, as you will have more distance to cover as you ride the corner and then make your approach. However, if your horse was inclined to run out, inexperienced, or you were up on time this might be your first choice. The second choice would be to jump the apex on a curve. In other words, you would rebalance as you approach the fence but make the turn over the fence rather than before it. To ride the fence this way you must be confident in your horse's ability to stick to the line you choose and not duck out the side at the last minute. You must also be confident that you can choose a good line. To ride a curving line over a fence, you must ride the curve with your outside aids, both leg and hand, and if necessary carry your

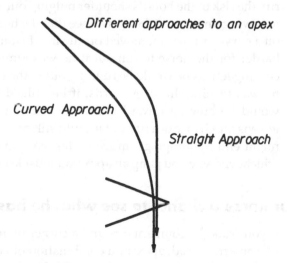

Figure 3.57 The two different options when jumping an apex.

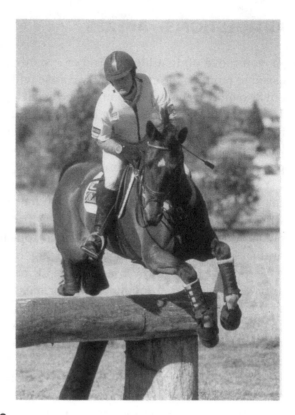

Figure 3.58

whip in the outside hand. If you just pull the inside rein to turn, you run the risk of the horse's shoulder bulging out with the rest of his body following. In Figure 3.58 you can see that the horse has jumped the apex on a curve but has not moved off the line I wanted to take. It would be harder for the horse to run out if he was jumping the same apex but curving left, as he would be running out in the opposite way to the way he was turning. In other words, if he bulged his outside shoulder it would be bulging toward the fatter end of the apex. Although this lessens the chance of a run-out it could still cause a problem because you might end up jumping a much wider fence than you had planned, so whichever way you jump an apex you must keep to your line.

Give your horse a chance to see what he has to do

If you walk the course and round a corner there is a technical complex like an arrowhead, apex, or a combination of both, remember that you can't expect the horse to look around the corner. Therefore when you come across this situation the straighter you have the horse the easier it will be for him to look in a straight line and assess what he is about to do. I also like to have my horses straight in their body, because I find it easier to control them. When you have them straight they should find it harder to slide a shoulder out or run out, so if you have a technical question or an apex it is a good idea to spend a few extra seconds turning a little wider, getting their body straighter and allowing them to see and assess the fence.

DOUBLE OF APEXES – A COMBINATION FENCE

In my opinion, combination fences tend to be the hardest for the horse and rider to negotiate as there is a lot to look at and do in a short space of time. At least the rider will have walked the course and know what is coming, but the horse has to make a lot of judgements in a few seconds. Hopefully the rider will be of some help, but ultimately it is the horse who picks his legs up. The training of the horse will play a big part in whether he manages to negotiate a combination fence successfully. Does he stay straight? Does he jump too big into the water but is still able to come back to the rider and stay on track? Does he stay in the same rhythm or is he stalling or rushing?

In the next two sequences of photos I jump a double of apexes which gives me two choices for my route through the fence. The horse must stay on whatever line I choose.

Faster and straighter

In Figures 3.59–3.61 I have ridden a straight line between the two fences, which means I will take three strides in between the elements. I came on a curved line then straightened before the first fence. This is the quickest route, but it does allow the horse more opportunity to run out of either apex so you must feel confident that he will stay on your chosen line.

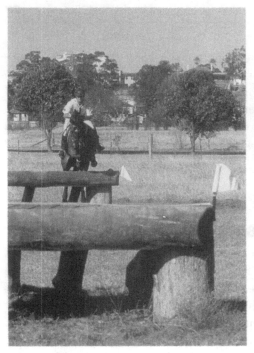

Figure 3.59

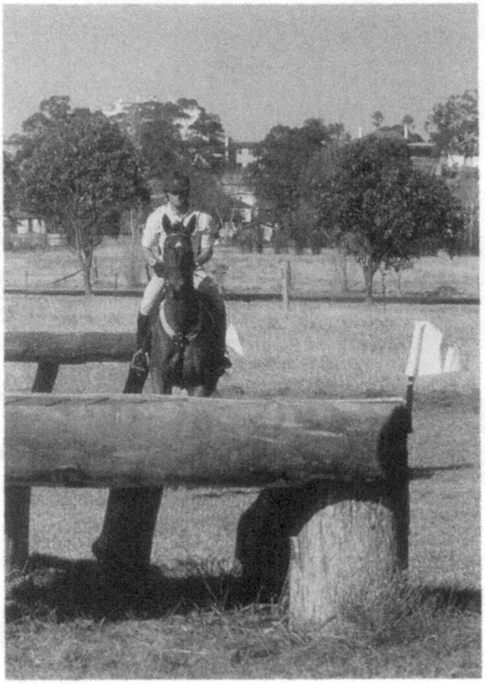

Figure 3.60

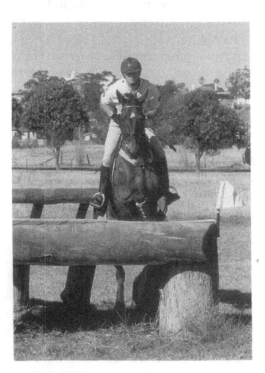

Figure 3.61

Slower and curved

In Figures 3.62–3.65 I have chosen to take a curving line between the two fences. This is the slower, but safer option, as it will allow me to jump each apex square onto the front rail which will lessen the chances of a run out, but will mean I have to take four strides in between the first and second elements. Whichever option I choose for this fence, the rebalancing would be about the same and I would still come in at the same sort of pace because I'm not actually riding a forward three strides or a holding four, I'm riding a different line with different distances.

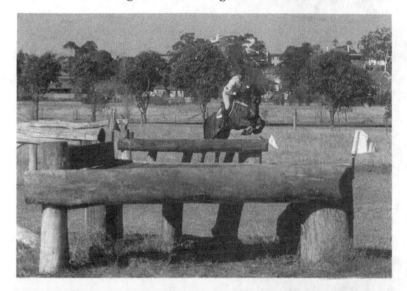

Figure 3.62

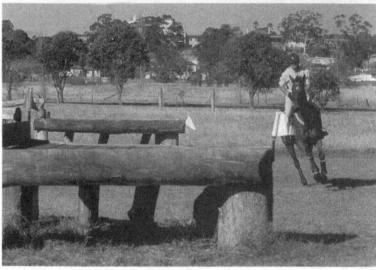

Figure 3.63

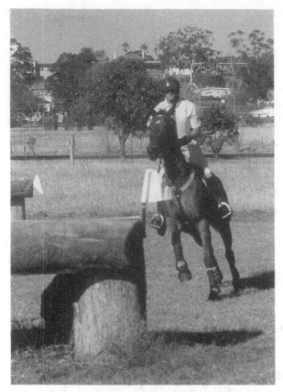

Figure 3.64

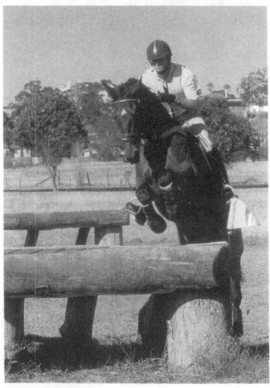

Figure 3.65

THE FINISH

I don't treat the finish any differently from the rest of the course. If you have been checking your watch you will know whether or not you are on time, and unless the finish is a considerable distance from the last fence not a lot will be gained from jumping the final fence and bolting to the finish flag. Many riders don't really think of what happens after you have gone through the finish, apart from those feelings of relief, euphoria, anguish or a mixture of all three. However, it is important to be aware of how you pull up. Bring your body into a more upright position so that the horse knows you want to slow down, and if necessary give a few half halts until he listens to you. Come back to trot and trot a straight line to check that the horse is feeling sound. Then slow down to walk and finally halt and jump off. For some combinations the finish is more of a lean back and pull, but in that instance the chances are that this combination has been the same through the whole course, so the finish will be no different. In those cases more training is needed to teach the horse that gallop is not the only pace.

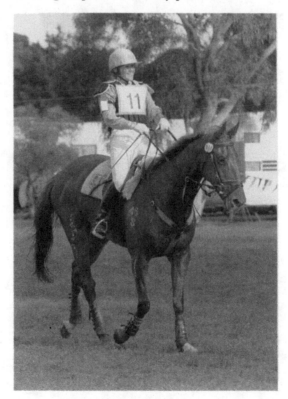

Figure 3.66 It's all about finishing with a happy rider and a happy horse.

Training for cross country in the arena

4

Training a horse for cross country is like training a horse to do anything else. Your instructions must be consistent, clear and correct. The horse cannot be expected to improve if you change your training methods from day to day, so you must decide what you are asking the horse to do, how you are going to ask him to do it, and follow it through. Showjumping can play a large part in cross country training. It will not only introduce your horse to various types of fence like planks and fillers, but also to all the decoration that goes along with a showjumping course, such as flower pots sitting beside fences. It can also help by getting the horse used to the different types of approaches needed for different fences. For example, an oxer will need to be approached in a stronger canter and the fence will open the horse up much more than an upright style fence, which will need to be approached in a steadier canter. Try to take your young horse to as many showjumping days as possible so that even before he starts his cross country training he will be quite comfortable with several types of fence.

Once your horse is jumping confidently over showjumps and has done some grid work you can start to include some cross country training in your work in the arena. Obviously the arena is flat, so you won't have the undulations that you would get on a cross country course, but nevertheless several exercises can be carried out which will help you when you ride your cross country round. I believe that all jumping exercises should encourage the horse to think quickly so he learns to assess a situation in a very short time and is not surprised by anything he might be asked to jump at an event.

MY THOUGHTS ON TRAINING

I want the horse to take off precisely where I want him to, and I will train him towards that. The horse is ultimately the one picking up his legs to get over a fence, and a precise rider will give him the best chance of getting over the fence safely. The horse will gain confidence if he is ridden well. If, in training, the horse jumps one fence a little big and gets a bit close to the next, there is a chance he will try to move slightly off line to give himself more space. To the horse this would seem a sensible thing to do, but the rider knows that after the second jump there is a third and then a fourth, and by going off the line at the second there is little chance of making it to the fourth. If, in training, I allow the horse to move sideways, he will learn to cheat by rolling his body, which is not good. I will teach the horse that if he does jump a bit big he will stay on the line, shorten a little and be neater in front when he comes to the second fence, and still be on line for the next two. On the whole, the horse will always try to cheat because he doesn't know what is coming up after a particular fence. No matter how precise you are, you will never take the horse's instinct to think away from him, but you can try to make his job easier.

The line of approach to a fence and your speed should determine how well you jump that fence. Whether you are jumping at an event or in the arena, it is important to focus on the fence you are about to jump. As you ride the turn in the arena before the exercise, make sure you turn and look towards where you are going. Once you are on a straight line keep focused on the fence until you have jumped it. Have a plan of how you are going to ride away from the fence: are you going to turn left or right, or stop on a straight line? Obviously, you might have to change the plan for some reason connected with the way you have jumped the fence, but don't just land in a heap and fall around the next corner as you will give yourself much more work to do when you rebalance your horse for the next approach.

Good riders make good horses
Good riders don't usually have just one good horse, they have several. This is because the better you ride, the nicer it is for the horse and the more he will enjoy his eventing and work with you, and consequently the better the result will be. The horse gains, or loses, his confidence from the rider. If a good rider makes a mistake, the horse will usually forgive him knowing that most of the time he gets it right. If a rider consistently makes mistakes, the horse is much less likely to forgive him. This is why it is so important to try to

become a better rider, because in doing that the job of riding will become easier because it will be easier for the horse and he will then start to help you.

THE BOUNCE

I never really train over bounce fences when I go cross country schooling, because if the horse makes a mistake he could hit a leg on a solid fence and get an unnecessary injury. Therefore I like to teach my horses how to jump bounce fences in the relative safety of the arena. In the arena you are also able to play with the distances of the bounce, teaching the horse to shorten or lengthen, as both skills will be necessary on the cross country course. Some horses find it quite difficult to jump through a short bounce, but plenty of practice using a small fence should soon give them the idea.

In Figure 4.1 the bounce is set at 3 metres (10 ft). Caro, who is relatively inexperienced, has not brought up her front legs very neatly but she has done enough to clear the fence. She has certainly not backed off the exercise, which is a good sign, and I would expect that with practice her technique should improve. Note how my body position stays quite balanced with a steady lower leg position throughout the two fences, allowing Caro to work out the exercise for herself without any interference from me.

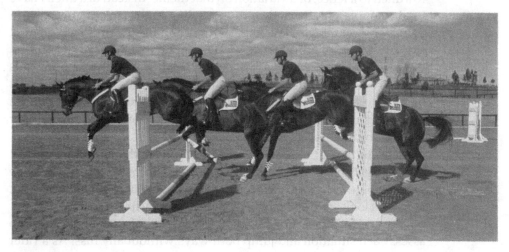

Figure 4.1

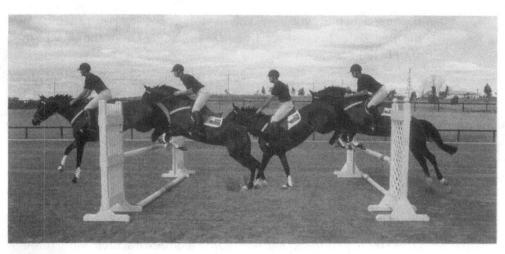

Figure 4.2

In Figure 4.2 I have moved the bounce out to 4.25 metres (14 ft) and you can see the difference in the shape that Caro has made between the shorter and longer distance. Here her frame is much more open and she jumps both fences quite easily

COFFIN OR SUNKEN ROAD

This exercise will replicate a coffin or sunken road fence, that is a fence to a ditch to a fence, or a variation on that theme. Instead of a ditch I have used a couple of rails on the ground, filling in the space between with planks to discourage the horse from putting his feet into the 'ditch'. I start off riding a vertical fence, landing and bouncing over the rails on the ground (Figure 4.3). The distance between the vertical and the rails is 3 metres (10 ft). You usually find the first time your horse sees the rails on the ground he will get a bit of a shock and probably won't make a very good jump. In Caro's case her shock made her jump quite big over the rails, but she did make a good shape.

Once the horse is jumping confidently over this exercise I turn it around so that the rails on the ground are jumped first and then the vertical (Figure 4.4). This will change the horse's focus from the vertical, as he will look at the ditch first. Some horses may find the exercise easier one way or the other. Either way it is just a case of training the horse to assess each situation and jump both ways without any fuss. As a rider you must be sure to look at the first element you are going to jump. For

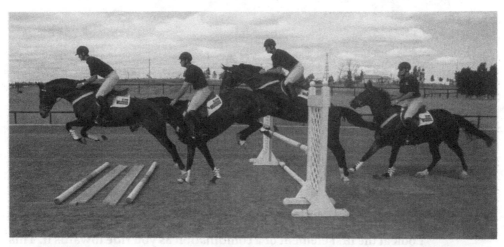

Figure 4.3

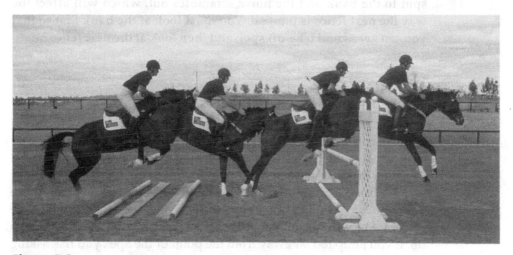

Figure 4.4

example, when you jump the ditch first you must come into the fence looking at the front rail of the ditch. If you look at the vertical you will find it difficult to get a good spot to the ditch.

After this exercise has been repeated a few times I add another vertical element to the combination so that I am jumping a vertical, bouncing the rails, and then have one stride of 6.7 metres (21 ft) to another vertical (Figure 4.5). The distances between the elements can be varied to teach the horse to shorten and/or lengthen.

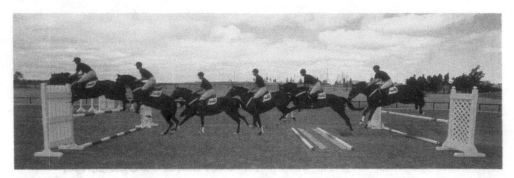

Figure 4.5

Where should I look?

Look at the first element of a combination as you ride towards it. This is often not done when riders are coming up a bank from water and have a fence just after the water. Because of this they don't get a good spot to the bank and the horse scrambles out, which will affect the way the next fence is jumped. You must look at the bank first so that you can get a good take-off spot, and then look at the next fence.

APEX TRAINING

Training over an apex or corner fences in the arena is very useful because you have more flexibility over the width and size of the corner than you would if you were cross country schooling. I have used a 44 gallon drum as one end of the corner with normal wings at the other end. I work on getting the horse to jump almost over the point of the apex or drum so if, in competition, the horse gets very close to the edge of a fence he will still jump it because that is what he has been trained to do. If you jump too far away from the point of the apex you risk asking your horse to jump what could be a very wide fence. This can be seen in Figures 4.6–4.8, where the horse has had to make an enormous effort to jump the fence. At the higher level of competition the angle of the apex is usually 90 degrees, so to be fair to your horse you have to jump the point – you have no choice.

In many respects jumping an apex is just like jumping an oxer, but of course there is always the chance of running out to the pointed end of the apex. You can see from Figure 4.9 that on Caro's first attempt at the apex she managed to dodge out of the corner. The next time round I made sure I kept a straighter line all the way in and held onto that line both up to and over the fence, and she jumped it well (Figure 4.10).

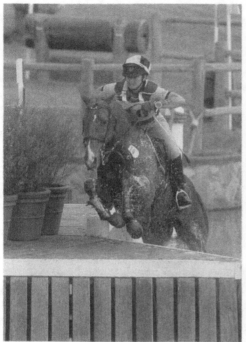

Figure 4.6

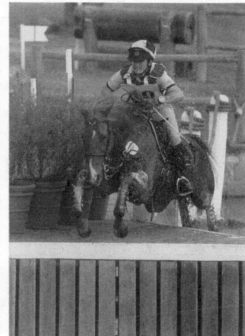

Figure 4.7

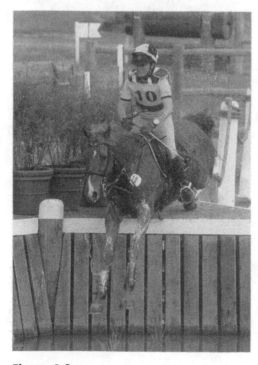

Figure 4.8

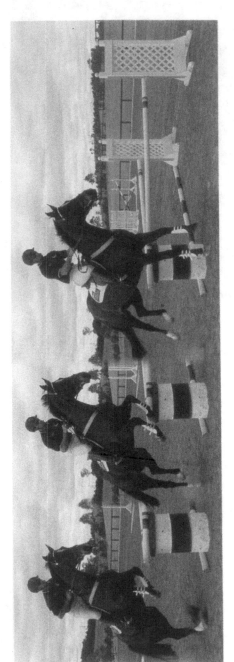

Figure 4.9

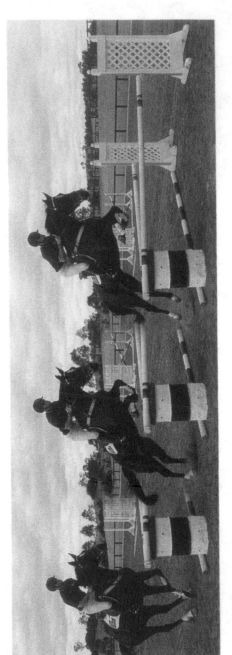

Figure 4.10

ARROWHEADS

Riding an arrowhead is similar to riding an apex in that the horse must jump exactly where you want him to. He must not move off the line you have chosen, and you must choose a good line. I start off using the 44 gallon drum on its side with a rail lying off either side of it to produce a funnel effect and assist the horse to be straight in his approach. Occasionally, the horse might be put off by the guiding rails, but generally they help the horse to focus on what you are asking him to do and the jump shouldn't be a problem.

In Figure 4.11 Caro jumps the drum but is a little wobbly as can be seen by the way she is leaning to her right underneath me. As I jump these fences I try to keep my body position totally focused on going straight.

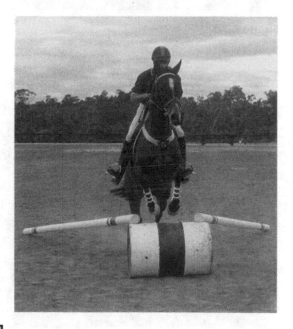

Figure 4.11

After jumping this a few times I will come into the fence from the other direction so that I am jumping the drum first before going into the spreading funnel (Figures 4.12, 4.13). This means that the horse loses the guidelines of the rails coming into the drum, but she does have the rails to keep her straight on the landing side. You can see in Figures 4.12 and 4.13 that without the funnel in, Caro has jumped the drum higher

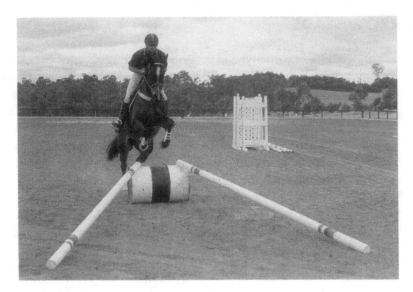

Figure 4.12

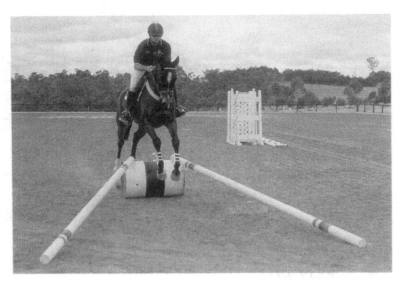

Figure 4.13

than previously. This is probably because she could see the rail on the other side of the drum.

Finally, I take the rails away completely and Caro jumps the drum on its own with a short rail acting as a ground line. The first time she attempts this she bulges out to the side at the last moment (Figure 4.14).

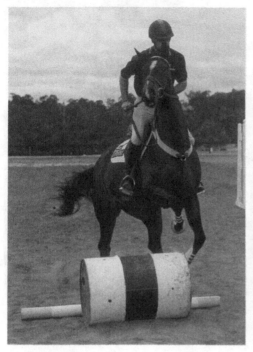

Figure 4.14

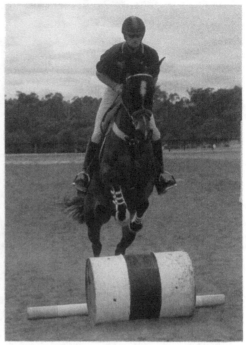

Figure 4.15

By the next attempt she has got the idea and jumps the drum straight and sensibly (Figure 4.15).

It will depend on your horse's level of training as to how quickly he will be able to work through these exercises. Asking a horse to do too much too quickly will only result in further problems along the track, so you must ensure that your horse is happy and confident at a certain level before you ask him to take the next step. Once the horse is confident with the exercise where the drum is on its side, we can make it harder by turning the drum to an upright position. Note that I have attached half a car tyre to the top of the drum, to protect the horse from any sharp edges. On the first attempt to this fence I used a standard length rail as a ground line and laid a short rail on top of the drum to help focus the horse's attention on the drum. You can see Caro is trying to have a good look at the drum when she jumps over it the first time and consequently doesn't make the best shape over the fence (Figure 4.16). She is also a little crooked in her body. After a few attempts, Caro is looking much more confident, her ears are pricked and she is looking ahead to see what is coming next. She has made a much better, rounder shape over the fence (Figures 4.17, 4.18).

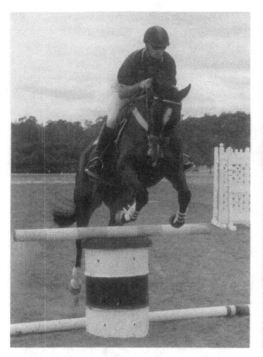

Figure 4.16

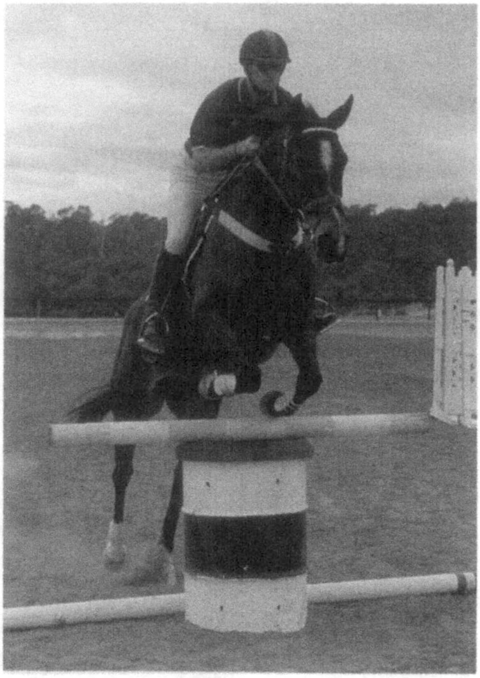

Figure 4.17

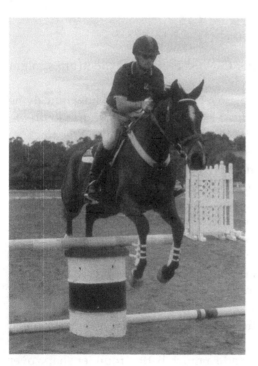

Figure 4.18

The final part of the exercise involves replacing the standard ground line with the short rail from the top of the drum and jumping the drum by itself. This is quite a difficult exercise for a horse and rider (Figures 4.19, 4.20). The rider must be very clear and correct about which line to take, and the horse must not waver off that line at all. We are asking the horse to jump a fence which is the same width as itself, so it requires a great deal of accuracy. If you are on an inexperienced horse, it could take several sessions before you reach this stage. For the more experienced horse, it is a good sharpening exercise to include in your routine. Because Caro was jumping the previous exercise quite happily she went on to jump the drum by itself very well. Note the position of her ears in Figure 4.19, which indicates that she was slightly apprehensive as she took off for the fence, but by the time she was in mid air (Figure 4.20) she was looking quite happy and confident.

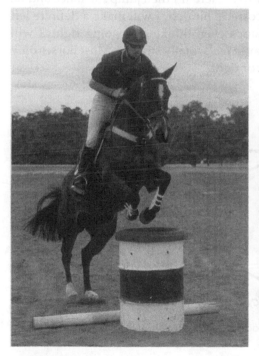

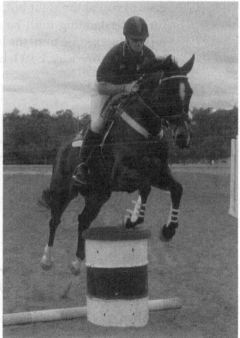

Figure 4.19   **Figure 4.20**

WHAT TO DO WHEN A HORSE RUNS OUT

You must turn your horse the opposite way to the way he has run out. For our example we shall use a run out to the right, so if your horse runs out this way you must turn him to the left. If you can, you should stop him before he goes past the fence, but this is not always possible. However, even if you have run past the fence you must still turn to the left. Using the left rein, take your horse back to the fence and take him out to the left before you make your next approach. It doesn't matter where you end up when you run out but you must turn him to the left (Figure 4.21). Do not allow him to go right, as this will only encourage him to run out the same way next time. If my horse is persistent in running out I won't just turn him left, I will turn him in some small circles to the left repeatedly until he starts to think about turning left himself. Sometimes you can be turning left but still feel the horse thinking right and his body wanting to go to the right. If this is the case, I keep turning until he brings all of his body to the left. If I then jump the fence and he goes to run to the right but corrects himself, I will make a definite left turn after landing until he stops even thinking of going right. I will repeat the exercise until the horse feels totally straight. Most horses only tend to run one way, be it left or right.

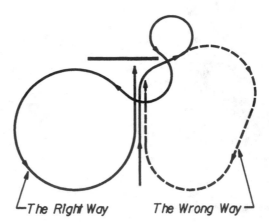

Figure 4.21   Turning to reapproach after a run out

Horse fitness **5**

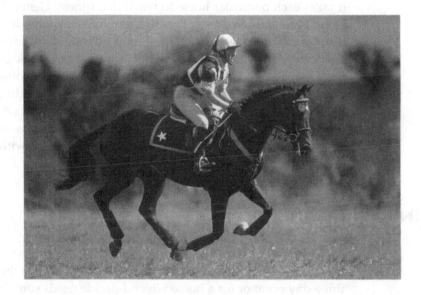

When you start a horse in his eventing career, the timing of his first event will be more related to his training rather than his fitness. If he has reached the required level of training for that event he will have done enough work to be fit enough to complete the event. To that extent I find it difficult to say my green horse will take, for example, 6 to 8 weeks before he is ready for his first one-day event, because in that time-frame I may not have taught him to jump well enough to tackle the cross country and showjumping courses. Therefore it all comes back to training.

In countries like Great Britain, many riders who are bringing horses into work, spend weeks doing hours of long slow road work in an

97

attempt to toughen up the horse's legs before they start doing any faster work. In Australia, I find this isn't necessary, because the horses are usually living out all the time and walking around on hard ground, so the joints in the majority of Australian horses actually need protecting from any undue jarring. In Great Britain, riders spend time searching for firmer ground to get out of the heavy deep going in which they often have to ride. In Australia, the opposite happens as we go looking for softer ground, which can often mean using the arena for the majority of the horse's work.

The ability to reach a certain level of fitness will vary with each horse. The breed, type and temperament will contribute to the length of time it takes each particular horse to reach that fitness. Generally speaking, I don't feel the need to gallop Thoroughbreds much, if at all, in the lead up to a one-day event. During their training I will have taken them cross country schooling, and I find that sort of work is enough as the Thoroughbred is bred to gallop anyway and quite often they have done some sort of racetrack work. However, if I'm riding more of a Warmblood type of horse, I might decide to do some fast work every fourth day as part of his training. I wouldn't ask the horse to do his first session of interval training until he was happily coping with at least half an hour of solid dressage work.

INTERVAL TRAINING

Before I start any interval training, I make a note of the horse's resting heart rate, as I will need this for a comparison later on. In the lead up to a three-day event or for a horse which I decide needs some gallop work, I will plan to do my faster work every fourth day, working on the programme set out here.

The first session comprises the following sequence:

- Working at a speed of 450–550 metres/minute, I canter the horse for 3 minutes.
- Walk the horse for 3 minutes
- Repeat the canter for 3 minutes
- Walk for 3 minutes
- Repeat the canter for 3 minutes
- The programme is complete.
- Four minutes after the last canter take the heart rate of the horse.
- After a further 10 minutes take the heart rate again. I would be looking for the heart rate to be a third of the way back to resting rate.

Example: Let's say the horse's resting heart rate is 36 beats/minute. Four minutes after the last canter the heart rate is 87 beats/minute. To check whether the horse is recovering quickly enough, do the following: $87 - 36 = 51$. For the horse to return to normal he has to drop 51 beats/minute from his highest heart rate reading. One-third of 51 is 17. If we subtract 17 from his highest heart rate reading (87) we obtain a figure of 70 beats/minute. Therefore if we measure the heart rate 14 minutes after the last canter and find it is below 70 beats/minute the horse is recovering at a reasonable rate. Of course, ideally you would be looking for the heart rate to be well under one-third of the way back to normal, but the recovery rate will depend on each individual horse.

If the figures show that the horse is recovering sufficiently quickly, I build up the time galloped at the next session. If he is not recovering as quickly as I would like, I will repeat the original session until he does improve.

With the horse who is recovering sufficiently, the sessions would increase by 1 minute each time. For example, at the second session I would work in 4 minute canters, still with 3 minutes in between each canter. If I increase the length of the canter sessions I would not increase the speed of the canter.

For a horse working towards his first novice (one star) three-day event I would expect to work up to cantering three, 6- or 7-minute sessions. For a more experienced horse aiming for his first advanced (three star) three-day event, I would like to build up to three 8- or 9-minute canters. The work depends very much on the horse you are riding, and you must treat each horse as an individual.

Try to carry out all your faster work on the best possible going. Hard ground will jar the horse's legs, and heavy going could cause the horse to strain a tendon or ligament, while uneven ground can damage the horse's joints.

Although I use the monitoring of heart rates as an indication of how fit a horse is, I also believe that feel plays an important part. The heart rate will usually confirm what I am already feeling, so it is important to be a thinking rider, not just in the dressage arena, but when you do your interval training as well. Think of how the horse feels underneath you. Is he remaining in balance or is he struggling with the pace? Is he keen to go again when you come to do your last canter or is he reluctant? If he is reluctant you will probably find his heart rate will reflect this, in that it will not be going down sufficiently quickly in the nominated time. If you follow the programme above, you should find the horse will get fit.

If he is struggling with the programme there might be an underlying problem, so consult your vet who will be able to advise you on the best plan of action.

OTHER METHODS OF GETTING FIT

Hill work

If you are lucky enough to have access to an uphill gallop, you will find you can cut down on the length of interval training and work on galloping up the hill. The amount of work done on the hill will depend on the length and severity of the incline, but you should be looking for a similar recovery rate as for the interval training.

Swimming

Although swimming is not a normal activity for a horse, it can be a great supplement in getting horses fit because it helps improve their aerobic fitness without putting any stress on their joints. Some horses take to swimming quite easily, whereas others will make no attempt to swim and nearly sink or panic. For this reason, the introduction should be made gradually and in a very safe situation where you know you are able to lead the horse out to dry ground if necessary. When you start to swim the horse I would recommend that the first session be a maximum of three 1 minute swims. Just as in gallop work, the heart rate of the horse must be taken so that a record can be kept on his progress.

TIME OFF

With an experienced horse who is being prepared for a three-day event, I don't find it necessary to give the horse a day off. However, they might work really well one day during the week and only need to be schooled for 20 minutes, so it's not as if they are working really hard seven days a week. Because most Australian horses live outside they can stretch their legs all day, so although they may only get lightly worked by their rider on one day they are still exercising themselves as they meander round the paddock. Horses confined to a stable for most of the time don't have that luxury, and therefore they tend to need more work in their training sessions.

I do tend to give the young horses a few days off after they have been to a one-day event, but I don't believe it is absolutely necessary to do that. There isn't usually as much pressure on young horses as there is on experienced horses so it doesn't matter if the young ones take it easy for a couple of days after an event. In fact, I think it is quite good for them mentally. However, if you have a particular problem at an event, you may choose to work on that problem on the days immediately following. Each situation is different and it's up to you to choose the best plan to adopt.

I work on a 12 week programme if I'm getting a horse ready for a three-day event and therefore the time off afterwards very much depends on when the next three-day event is planned for. Obviously, if the horse has an injury he will require the appropriate time to recover, and then I might bring him into work a little earlier than the normal 12 weeks to give him a little bit longer to get fit. I believe you need to have a good plan for each horse, but as horses are renowned for going lame just at the wrong time, you also have to be very adaptable around that plan.

HOW CAN YOU TELL IF YOUR HORSE IS GETTING TIRED?

If you follow this programme, your horse should get fit and be able to cope with his eventing. However, there are always situations where, for various reasons, the horse may begin to tire on the cross country course. Perhaps the ground is particularly heavy and the horse has struggled with the conditions, or maybe the course has proved to be quite tough and the horse has put in a big effort. Either way, it is important to realise what it feels like if your horse starts to tire and what action to take. If the horse I'm riding is getting harder to rebalance, feeling a little uncoordinated, or simply not going on when I ask him to, there is a fair chance he is starting to get tired. If that is the case, and depending how far round the cross country course I am, I might have to change my plan of how I ride the rest of the course. I would certainly be trying to get the horse home as smoothly as possible without making abrupt adjustments to his way of going. Obviously, I would still rebalance before each fence, but without breaking his rhythm too much and because I wouldn't be travelling as fast I wouldn't have to rebalance as much. When the horse is tired he may not be able to react as quickly as normal to certain situations, or he may not have his usual scope. Because of this it's not a good idea to take off a long way out from a fence, as he would find it more difficult to make the distance over the jump.

It is important to recognise that there is a difference between a tired horse and a lazy horse. Some horses need to be encouraged to gallop on a cross country course simply because it is not in their nature to gallop. This comes back to the training of the horse, where he should be taught to gallop consistently during interval training, and, of course, knowing what is normal for each horse.

Horse management

GENERAL

The horse can only perform at his best if he is fit and well, so good horse management plays a vital role in your horse's eventing career. As you put hours of training into your horse, it would be foolish not to look after him properly before, during and after each event.

KNOW YOUR HORSE

Good horse management starts at home, where you must take the time to get to know the various quirks of your horse. Is he a worrier? Does he keep condition on easily, or does he lose weight quickly if he gets stressed? Is he a bit stiff when you first start riding him, or does he feel really sound from the word go? Get to know every lump and bump on his body, his legs in particular. That way you will notice something new straight away and be able to treat it accordingly.

STICK TO ROUTINE

Horses are creatures of habit and are more likely to do well if they are kept to a routine, so try to feed your horse at the same time every day. This is especially important if the horse is kept in a stable, or for a nervous type of horse who will lose weight just worrying that his food has not arrived at the same time as normal.

PROTECTION

The legs of event horses are under a lot of strain because of all the galloping and jumping involved in eventing. Therefore their legs must be well looked after if you want your horse to compete for several years whilst avoiding major injury. Prevention is better than cure, and you can help to avoid an injury by using boots or bandages on your horse during all his work sessions. As well as acting as a layer of protection for a horse who might brush his legs together as he works, the boots will also protect the legs against any injury caused by a leg scraping a fence.

I prefer to use boots, as they are easier and quicker to put on than bandages. If you choose to use bandages, you must use some form of padding underneath them, and great care must be taken not to put them on too tightly and that they do not come off during training or competition.

For some horses, it can be just as important to protect their legs even when they are not being ridden. Horses who live out and are, on occasion, inclined to gallop in their paddock may need the protection of boots when they are turned out because this will lessen the chance of them cutting into themselves. Be very careful in your choice of boots, as a boot which is being left on for several hours must not rub the leg or cause it to sweat and heat up. Skin conditions can be caused or made worse by using a boot that heats up the skin. I use a brushing boot with sheepskin on the inside. I find they do not rub, the sheepskin allows the horse's leg to breathe and therefore it doesn't get too hot. In an Australian summer I would much rather not put anything on horses' legs as they undoubtedly would sweat, but the pros and cons have to be added up and then you can make an informed decision. Horses who live inside and whose legs tend to fill up may benefit from wearing bandages, as they will help with the circulation.

LOOKING AFTER LEGS

After any hard and fast work, such as a gallop session, a one-day or three-day event, I follow the same routine of using iced water on my horse's legs. I find ice the best treatment as it is cheap and simple to use, and helps to reduce blood flow to any possible injury sites. Applying ice or iced water to the leg can be done in various ways, but whichever way you choose, be sure that ice never comes into direct contact with the horse's skin as it will damage that area. I use a pair of rubber tub ice boots, which go up and over the horse's knees, and are filled with iced water.

Although initially the horse might take a little while to get used to the boots, once they have had them on a few times they aren't usually too worried by them. After a gallop session I might only use the boots for one 20 minute session after which, if the legs remain cool with no obvious hot spots, I would be happy that everything is fine. If a particular spot heats up, make sure you take note of where that area is, so that after your next gallop session you can check that same area. Be aware that if your horse has sustained a rub, the use of ice will cause that rubbed area to heat up, so put some petroleum jelly over the rubbed area before you apply ice to the rest of the leg. After a cross country round I use the boots as many times as necessary to get the legs back to normal. If after the first treatment the legs don't heat up too quickly, I leave the boots off for 20 minutes and then put them back on for a further 20 minutes. If the legs start to heat up after 5 minutes, following the initial 20 minutes treatment, I put the boots back on for a further 20 minutes and then reassess. Every horse and each situation is different, but barring any major problems I would expect to use the boots three or four times after the cross country of a three-day event, or until I'm happy that the legs are back to normal. Be sure to add fresh ice to the boots each time they are used, as the first ice will have melted a little with the heat of the horse's legs. If the legs are still hot after using the boots for several sessions, consult your vet, as there may be a serious problem. There are several ice boots on the market which have pockets in them which can work really well, so you are not just limited to using the tub ice boots.

Ice or ice packs can be very useful on other areas of the horse which may have sustained an injury, a stifle for example. In this situation wrap the ice in a towel and simply hold it on the affected area for 20 minute sessions.

RAPID OR AGGRESSIVE COOLING

It is very important after any fast work, or indeed after any sort of work where the horse gets hot, that his temperature is brought back to normal as quickly as possible. For this I use the now common practice of rapid cooling.

It has been discovered that the most effective way to cool a horse is to apply cold water to the horse's body and then immediately scrape it off. The importance of scraping the water off quickly cannot be over emphasised because water left on the body for too long will simply heat up, blocking the horse's most efficient cooling system, his skin. Rapid cooling is best carried out by two or three people, so that the continuous action of applying water and scraping it off can be carried out. If the horse, and the weather, are extremely hot, the addition of some ice to the washing water can be helpful. Hosing the horse is another option which works well as long as the water is scraped off before hosing again.

SHOEING

Although your horse should be well shod at all times, it is especially important that your horse's shoes are in good condition for a competition. A loose shoe, or even a risen clench, could cause an injury to another leg when you are galloping or jumping, or even warming up for your dressage test.

Make sure the farrier you use is registered, because if the horse is not correctly shod it can lead to all sorts of other problems, including strains, over-reaches and stress on joints. It is worth remembering that when a horse is shod, we automatically make his feet stay on the ground a little longer than those of an unshod horse. Therefore, if we let the shod horse go too long between shoeings, the toe will become too long and cause all sorts of complications. Keeping the toe short and rolling it may help to soften the way the horse's foot leaves the ground, which will cause less strain to the leg. Discuss your horse's needs with your farrier who will be able to advise you concerning the best type of shoes for your horse.

Horse types

7

There are no set rules when it comes to looking for an event horse. Personal preference, the temperament, and whether you actually like and get on with the horse can be the most important factors for some people, especially if you are a one horse owner. After all why would you want to spend a considerable amount of time and effort with a horse you didn't like? However, when you go beyond personal preference, there are several other factors that should be taken into consideration as you go on the search for your event horse.

CONFORMATION

Conformation is the shape of the horse and the way he is put together. Conformation is important as it will affect the horse's ability to carry out the job you want him to do. Beauty is not important, although you do tend to find that a horse with good conformation is usually a good looking horse, but not necessarily a pretty horse. The horse must be well proportioned with nothing looking out of place. Occasionally, you see a horse with great conformation from the shoulder up but the legs look as if they belong to another horse, either because they are very long or very short – they just don't match with the rest of the body. As a rough guide if you stand back and look at the horse you should be able to visualise his body, from the point of his shoulder to his rump, fitting into a square shape. If the square is more of a rectangle, it points to the horse having a long back and, although this isn't usually a major problem, it can make it harder for the horse to work in a correct outline. Another common problem is a horse with an underdeveloped neck and/or a seemingly big head. The underdeveloped neck may, over time, develop into a better shape, but it would be fair to say that the head will stay the same size. However, certainly for the novice rider, a horse with either of these problems should not be dismissed too quickly as he may turn out to have the kindest temperament and give you years of enjoyment.

A horse with a neck which doesn't come up from the withers will always be inclined to go on the forehand. He may eventually build up muscles which will help him carry himself, but it is preferable to have a horse with a good connection between his neck and the rest of his body.

The legs and feet are obviously some of the most important parts of the horse. The joints, tendons and ligaments in the horse's legs have to withstand enormous stresses and strains during jumping, while the feet have to endure various ground conditions, including wet, heavy, dry or hard. The legs should be in proportion with the rest of the horse's body and, as much as possible, need to have correct conformation. The leg should be straight with the joints sitting in the leg correctly and, again, nothing should look out of place. Regarding the front legs, a horse with a longer forearm and shorter cannon bone should be less prone to soundness problems than a horse with the opposite attributes. This is because the horse with longer cannon bones will also have longer tendons which are more prone to strain injury than shorter ones. For the back legs, the muscle above the horse's hock, the gaskin, should be well developed, as it will be working with the hock when the horse jumps and therefore needs to be strong. All this aside, there are several event horses at the top level who don't possess the greatest legs, but for whatever reasons they stay sound and keep on going.

When you stand back and look at the horse as a whole, it is amazing to think those four relatively small feet bear the entire weight of the horse. The feet are the first things to take the full weight of the horse on landing after a fence, so they must be as close to the correct shape as possible for that particular horse. The hooves should be round and large, and in proportion with the horse. Small feet tend to be more upright and this can cause jarring of the horse's legs, whereas overly large feet tend to be flat which can lead to bruising of the sole simply because the sole is too close to the ground. Overly large sloping feet can also put more strain on the tendons. It is important that the two front feet look the same, as uneven feet will lead to more pressure on one foot or the other, and when the pastern and fetlock joints are subjected to more strain so are the tendons and ligaments.

The horse's stride and consequent paces will be determined by the way the legs are set onto the body. Good paces are helpful, but certainly not essential, if you only intend to event at a low level. However, if you aspire to partake in top class eventing, and given the ever improving standard of dressage, you need to make sure your potential event horse has good quality paces with a good length of stride and a good rhythm. Look for a horse who seems to find it easy to trot in the same rhythm, be it on a straight line or going round a corner. The canter should look effortless, smooth and balanced, with no scuttling around corners. Sometimes nerves, stress or lack of balance can disguise a horse's paces, and this is often seen in an ex-racehorse who is being trained to event. In this case, the decision of how good the paces are will relate to the horse's temperament, how trainable he is and whether he will relax enough to let his true paces show through. Education will play a large part in how your horse goes in many ways, but if your horse has a good temperament and wants to learn, that will be a great help for all your training.

BREED

Horses which are bred to gallop will obviously find it easier to reach a higher level of eventing than those horses who were bred for other purposes, simply because their breeding and conformation will make the job easier. However, at a lower level the gallop may not be so important as other attributes, so I think it is very much an individual choice as to the type of horse you decide to event. It comes back to the fact that personality is more important to a lot of people than a specific breed. One of the most important attributes of the horse, be it Thoroughbred or stock horse, is its brain, and I don't believe you can label a breed with a certain brain. For example, many people believe Thoroughbreds to be very highly strung, but personally I don't find that. I think it depends on the individual horse. You cannot put a brain on a breed – not *all* Thoroughbreds are highly strung, nor are all Warmbloods submissive and quiet. Whatever breed you choose, you must remember the job you want the horse to do. The three-day event horse needs a lot of stamina, speed and toughness, whereas an event horse who will be running round a few pre-novice events every year will not need those qualities to the same degree. In Australia, the majority of event riders compete on ex-racehorses simply because they are relatively cheap to buy and easily available. However, this does not mean you should discount a cross-breed horse. In Europe many Thoroughbreds have been crossed with a draught breed such as Clydesdale, Percheron or Irish, with great results. Coloured horses also have their place in eventing as many people find them easy to get on with, because they seem to have plenty of common sense. With the ever improving standard of eventing dressage, many riders are opting for a Thoroughbred crossed with Warmblood in the hope of getting a better set of paces together with softness.

SOUNDNESS

Soundness is very much related to conformation, and horses with good legs and feet stand a much better chance of staying sound. However, there is also the pain threshold to take into account. Just like humans, different horses will put up with the same pain in different ways. A tough horse will keep going even though he has banged a leg, whereas another horse might suffer the same injury and hardly put the foot to the ground. Toughness isn't something which necessarily comes with a certain breed, it comes as part of the personality of that horse. When you take an initial look at a potential horse, ask the owners to trot him in a straight line and a small circle as this should show up any abnormalities in their way of going. If you decide to go further with the purchase of the horse, make sure that a thorough vet check is carried out. The soundness of a horse can also go together with the horse management skills of the person who looks after that horse. Many horses who have had minor, niggling problems have managed to stay sound thanks to good management. This could range from the treatment of legs after cross country to the fitness preparation of the horse.

SIZE

To be able to event officially, the horse must be over 148 cm high (14.2 $\frac{1}{4}$ hh), beyond which it is really the scope and talent of the horse that will determine how well he goes. There have been many great small horses over the years who have made it to the top level of eventing, including Mark Todd's dual gold Olympic horse Charisma who stood just 160 cm high (15.3 hh). Some people find small horses a little sharper with their legs over fences, while others prefer the feel of a big horse. Again it comes down to personal choice and what you feel comfortable riding.

TEMPERAMENT

The temperament and attitude of the horse will play a vital role in how well he succeeds as an event horse. The horse must be trainable and able to work with you. He must also be calm enough to deal with the stresses and excitement of competition. It's not much fun to put in hours of work at home only to find your horse reverts back to being a racehorse when he goes to an event. Of course, this might happen with the ex-racehorse on his first couple of outings to an event, but a horse with a trainable temperament will start to realise that going out can mean other things apart from racing. This is where intelligence comes into play. A horse with a good level of intelligence should make the rider's job a little easier. When you purchase your new horse there is a fair chance you will ride in a slightly different way from the previous owner. The intelligent horse and rider will recognise this and work out the differences during training. For example, a horse may have been taught to canter purely with a push from the outside leg, while you give the canter aid with a push from the inside leg. An intelligent horse shouldn't take too long to figure out what you want and switch to the new aids.

Take the time to understand your horse so you can work at making him the best possible competitor he can be. Ask yourself some questions: Does your horse concentrate or get easily distracted? Does he stay focused on the cross country course looking for the next fence, or is he always surprised when he is faced by it? Addressing all these things will go towards making the most out of your event horse.

REQUIREMENTS AND ABILITY

When you are looking for your event horse, you should have a clear picture in your mind of what you expect that horse to be able to do for you. Are you looking for a horse who will take you around some Pony Club courses and perhaps a few pre-novice tracks, or are you looking for a horse with the potential to go around a four star track? What will be the most important thing to you about this horse: the shape it makes over a fence or the fact that it has an easy going temperament and won't worry if you aren't able to ride every day? Be realistic in your expectations and those of your potential horse and, who knows, you might be as lucky as Australia's Wendy Shaefer who bought Sunburst while she was in the Pony Club to do Pony Club events and ended up partnering him to a gold medal at the Atlanta Olympics.

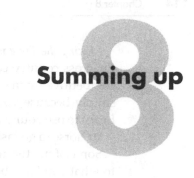

Summing up

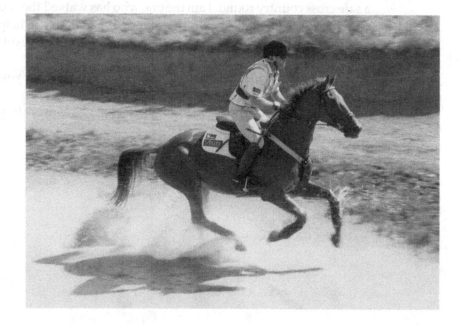

Eventing should be enjoyable for both horse and rider. The better you can train your horse and yourself, the more enjoyable it will be. I consider rebalancing the horse and keeping your eye on the fence to be two of the most important aspects of cross country riding. Of course, there are many other important points to consider when you head off around a course, but looking at each fence and rebalancing before each fence will help to put you and your horse in a safer situation. Train your horse to rebalance, and train yourself to look at the fence and choose a good take-off spot. Eventing safely comes down to a matter of choice and that is what I have tried to explain in this book.

Making the Time is not just about riding safely, it is also about riding the cross country course in the most efficient way so that you can be competitive by making the time. It is frustrating to lose a competition simply because you didn't choose the best route around the course. Learn to use your watch to your advantage so that you never have to ask your horse to go faster than necessary.

Some of my thoughts on riding cross country may be a little different to what you have been taught in the past, but it has to be remembered that cross country courses have changed considerably over the past 10 years, with far more technical questions now being asked. I believe the way I train my horses will give them and me the best chance of jumping a safe cross country round. I am the one who has walked the course and who then asks my horse to jump the fences, so I will try to help him as much as possible by riding well and using the techniques explained in this book.

The better you ride, the more advantageous it will be for your horse, and the easier your job will become.

I hope you and your horse go on to enjoy many safe years of eventing.

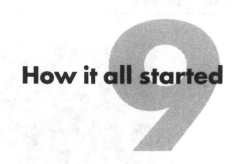

How it all started

I was born in 1964 in a small town called Mundubbera, Queensland. We moved to the slightly larger town of Gladstone, still in Queensland, when I was around 3 years old and we stayed there until the bank I was working for at the time transferred me to Brisbane. Neither of my parents were really 'horsey', although my dad, Brian, rode during his work mustering cattle. When I was around seven, dad took me along to a rally day at the local Calliope (the next town to Gladstone) Pony Club. I had never even sat on a horse or pony before, but it looked quite fun and when dad asked if I would like to go to Pony Club I said 'Sure, why not', and happily went along with the idea. As I didn't have my own pony when I first went to Pony Club, I rode a friend's pony and then, thanks to some friends of the family, dad managed to acquire a pony for me called Candy. Although she was lovely to people and basically nice to ride, she used to double barrel kick every horse or pony which came within a mile of her. Because of this I was always put at the end of any ride and had to spend all my time avoiding the other horses, which meant I didn't enjoy the most sociable of times in my early Pony Club days. However, I must have enjoyed riding enough, because about a year later I was still going to Pony Club but had nearly outgrown Candy and needed something not just bigger but a non-kicking version, and that's when I started riding Clyde. Clyde had originally been acquired for my sister, Paula, but because he bucked quite a bit he was quickly passed on to me. When he wasn't bucking he was really quite good, but I was falling off much more than I would have liked, so when I was around eight, Clyde found a new home and along came Gypsy, a 13.2 hh skewbald.

Gypsy was an amazing pony and together we won hundreds of ribbons (Figure 9.1). We took part in all the various classes at Pony Club, although you have to remember dressage wasn't really around in those

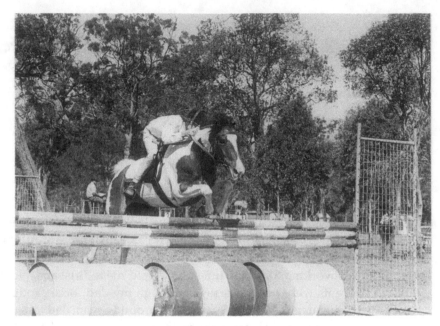

Figure 9.1 Gypsy and I won hundreds of ribbons together.

days so the term 'on the bit' meant absolutely nothing to me. We did jumping, sporting and rider classes, and when we were at a show where there was an overall point score winner at the end of the day I usually had a pretty good chance of winning. I did a little bit of Pony Club eventing with Gypsy because, in those days (around the mid-1970s) in central Queensland, there wasn't really any other kind of eventing available for younger people. I became really fond of Gypsy and, although I outgrew her in a few years, we kept her with us so she could see out her days in her own paddock.

When I was about fifteen and had grown too big for my 13.2 hh Gypsy, I moved on to a part Quarter horse called 76 whose name came from his brand of seven over six, not very original I know. 76 was, it has to be said, fairly untalented and, although I did try to showjump and event him we weren't terribly successful, which didn't impress me much. At this stage it really didn't matter to me whether I was taking part in jumping, sporting or rider classes, but I *did* want to win and certainly didn't enjoy losing. I soon decided it was time to call it quits with 76 and he was sold on to someone who, hopefully, didn't want to win as much as I did. The next horse to come along was a 7 year old ex-racehorse, straight off the track at Gladstone, whom I named Radical.

Radical

Dad, in the mid-1970s, was working as a horse/cattle auctioneer. When Radical, as he came to be known, went through his sale ring, dad thought he was a good type and put in a bid of $250 for him. Someone else put in a higher bid of $275, so dad thought he had missed out. However, the cheque for $275 bounced and because dad had been the next bidder in line he was offered the horse for his original bid of $250, so the ex-racehorse came to us after all. Radical certainly wasn't radical, in fact he was a wonderfully quiet horse, with good looks, really good movement and a very careful jumper. It is only now, looking back, that I realise just how good he was. At the age of 16 years I started Pony Club eventing Radical, and doing a little bit of dressage, although it would be fair to say I still didn't know what I was doing as I was mostly self taught with a little bit of Pony Club instruction thrown in. As I started to compete more with Radical I realised that if I was going to get anywhere I needed some help from someone outside the Pony Club. To that end I started to make the long 8 hour journey to Brisbane to have the occasional flat-work lesson with dressage instructor Ron Patterson who had been introduced to me by a friend who was also having lessons with him. As you can imagine, with that length of journey I didn't have many lessons, but my parents were always very supportive and dad would clock up hours of driving as he took Radical and me all over Queensland so that we could compete. My older sister Paula also rode, but was more into hacking and showing rather than eventing. Around the same time as I started to do more competing, Paula, who wasn't riding a particularly talented horse at the time, decided to move on to other things.

In the late 1970s and early 1980s when I was eventing Radical, the sport of 'official' eventing in Central Queensland was still in its very early days. We had to travel for hours just to get to an event and when you finally got there the cross country course usually consisted of a very dry paddock with several spindly looking fences built by good humoured volunteers trying to do the best they could. The 'theme' back in those days was certainly the natural look. If the paddock happened to have a natural gully there was often a fence placed at the top and bottom of the slope which, looking back now, was really quite hazardous, but we all survived, and from those humble beginnings the sport of eventing in Australia started to grow. Because of the lack of 'official' events, Pony Club eventing was very popular and I was lucky that within a few of our local Pony Clubs we had some pretty talented riders to compete against. Riders like sisters Prue Barrett (nee Cribb) and Felicity Cribb,

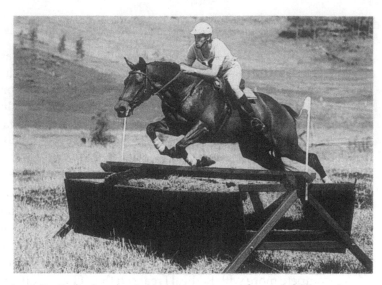

Figure 9.2 Radical and me taking part in one of our early three-day events at Kooralbyn.

brothers Mark and Greg Watson, and Maxine Jensen were all local riders who went on to represent either their state or indeed their country, so competition, even at that Pony Club level, was fierce. When I was around seventeen I won the Pony Club state one-day event and the National Pony Club one-day event with Radical, so I thought I was going alright, but it wasn't until I rode at my first 'official', non-Pony Club event that I realised I really still had an awful lot to learn.

That first 'official' event was a pre-novice three-day event at Kooralbyn in Queensland (Figure 9.2). Obviously, it would have been better to start at a one-day event, but with the shortage of events in general you couldn't be too choosy, so when Kooralbyn came along, off we went. It was certainly a shock to the system for both horse and rider, because I really had no idea of what a three-day event was all about. Luckily, several of my friends were in the same boat so we all tried to help each other. The camaraderie between all the competitors at Kooralbyn was great, and that camaraderie is one of the reasons I still love the sport today. In the event itself I got time penalties on phase C because I had no idea that if you finished phase B early, which I did, you then had to finish phase C that bit earlier. I just thought you had to finish phase C on the time stated on your time sheet. However, I have never made that particular mistake again. I didn't do terribly well at Kooralbyn, but I was quite philosophical about it and decided the only way to get better was just to keep trying, which I did.

When I left school, I started doing the responsible thing. For me, this was working in the local bank. When I was around twenty I was transferred to Brisbane, which was wonderful because I saw Brisbane as the eventing mecca of Australia. This was probably because I had always lived miles away from any 'official' events, and around the Brisbane area there was so much more going on which meant more events and at least a bit less travelling. I started to do more eventing and, although I wasn't hugely successful, I was good enough to get onto the Queensland state team where, luckily for me, Wayne Roycroft was the coach. Meeting Wayne and his wife Vicky turned out to be one of the best things that could have happened for me and my eventing career. After having some lessons with Wayne, I started to feel I was actually learning something and really understanding what it meant to ride a horse rather than just be a passenger. Thanks to Wayne's help, Radical and I started to clock up some good results, including our first three-day event win at Kooralbyn CCI** in 1987. After that win I decided to tackle my first CCI***, at Werribee in Melbourne, Victoria. Wayne suggested I should come and stay for a few weeks at his yard on the way to Melbourne, not only to give me some lessons but also to break the journey as the trip from Brisbane to Melbourne would take a couple of days in total. So I took some unpaid leave from the bank and headed off to Wayne and Vicky Roycroft's property at Mount White, just north of Sydney.

During those weeks of training, Radical was not looking 100% level and the decision was taken to abandon any thoughts of taking him to Melbourne. Radical never really came sound enough to three-day event, but I did manage to do some showjumping with him with some success. During those weeks at Wayne's he suggested I might like to stay and train with him, so I never went back to the bank and ended up staying at Mount White from 1987 to 1990. This proved to be such a great learning experience for me that without it I very much doubt if I would be where I am today – I owe a lot to both Wayne and Vicky Roycroft.

Patch of Silver

Whilst at Mount White, I got to ride Patch of Silver, owned by the Roycrofts. He was not an easy horse, which was probably why I was given him to ride – no one else wanted him! During the 3 years I spent at Mount White, Silver and I managed to achieve some results that were good enough to put us on a Trans Tasman team, and we were also long listed for the Seoul Olympics in 1988. The selection trial for Seoul was Melbourne CCI*** and although Silver jumped all the big complex fences, he stopped at a pathetic little drop, so needless to say we didn't get picked to go to Seoul.

Erimbula Bright Beacon

At Mount White, I not only had the advantage of learning from two of Australia's best riders, it also gave me the opportunity to meet various people who would go on to become, in some way, part of my future with horses. One of those people was Jane Bailey. Jane had bought a horse off the track called Erimbula Bright Beacon, otherwise known as BB. She competed BB for a while and then sold him on to Michelle Luff who rode him to advanced level. After getting married, Michelle decided she didn't want to compete at that level any more, so in preparation for selling BB, I was asked to ride and compete him for a while. BB was a lovely horse and after a couple of one-day events I took him to Gawler CCI*** in 1991. One of the members of the ground jury that year was Reiner Kilmke and when he placed me first after my dressage test I really felt that I had at last grasped the concept of dressage, or at least dressage on BB. However, from a good result on dressage day, the event went downhill thanks to some horrendously stormy weather conditions. The sky was so dark on cross country day that car headlights had to be shone on the fences just so that the riders and horses could see where they were going! By the time I went out on the cross country course it was already pretty dark and when I got to fence three, a sunken road complex, I had no idea of what I was about to jump into. I soon discovered that the whole landing side of the ditch had been washed down into the ditch itself, leaving the last vertical element sticking out of the ground. As BB tried to jump the ditch there was nothing for him to land on and he ended up straddling the vertical. By this stage I had collected hundreds of time penalties, but as BB came out of the whole experience uninjured I thought I might as well continue and we went on to jump the rest of the course without a problem. The sunken road fence was removed from the course following this incident. I have to admit it was pretty scary jumping the second-to-last fence which was a big bank, because although I knew where the fence was, I really couldn't see it – BB was such a brave horse to keep going. At the end of the day most of my time penalties were taken away as the ground jury felt the problems we had suffered at the sunken road were really not my fault. We finished the event in third place, a performance good enough to get us shortlisted for the 1992 Barcelona Olympics.

These days, Australian riders who are shortlisted to go to Europe in preparation for an Olympics or World Equestrian Games receive a great deal of help, both financial and practical, from the Australian Equestrian Federation. However, back in 1992 you were expected to fend for yourself once you arrived in the UK. Luckily for me, BB's original owner Jane Bailey, together with her husband John, had moved from Australia to the UK and were living in Herefordshire. John and Jane kindly offered to put us up, and after doing a couple of one-day events we headed off over the channel to Saumur, France, to take part in the CCI***. Saumur was a lovely event and I can remember riding round the roads and tracks thinking what a beautiful part of the world in which to hold a three-day event. I enjoyed a great weekend and came within 0.2 points of winning Saumur, but had to be content with second place, which I was still pretty pleased about.

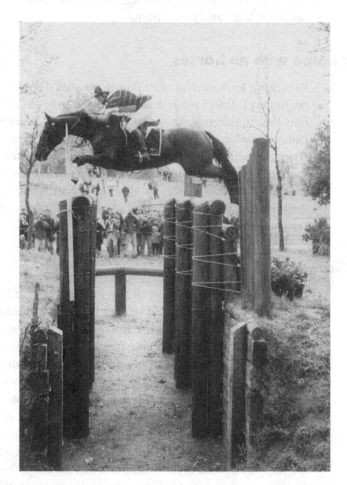

Figure 9.3 On our way to coming second at Saumur CCI*** in 1992 with Erimbula Bright Beacon.

We were named on the team for Barcelona and things were looking good. But as in most things with horses, you can never be too sure of anything, and the day we went into team training BB went lame with corns in his feet. He certainly didn't have the best feet in the world, but at home in Australia I had always managed to keep them in good shape. However, no matter what we tried in the UK nothing seemed to help, so one day we were heading for Barcelona and the next we weren't. The same day BB went lame, Karen, my fiancée, arrived from Australia and I had to tell her the sad news. We both decided to go to Barcelona anyway and support the other Australian riders and although I was obviously disappointed not to be riding it was good to watch my team mates win a gold medal. When we got back from Barcelona we assessed BB's situation and decided that, at his age, he should stay in England so he was retired at John and Jane's home.

Back home with no horses

Returning to Australia after Barcelona was depressing from the standpoint that I didn't really have any nice horses to ride. The only horse I had that was remotely near top level was a Warmblood × polo pony called Handel, and he became my three star eventer which he really struggled with. He could do quite a nice dressage test and jumped fairly well, but he really couldn't gallop and always found the time hard to make. Karen and I, who by this stage had set up a yard of our own, decided that we needed to find some good horses, which in turn meant we needed to find some good owners.

Tim Game

I have come to know most of my owners via my teaching or through friends of friends. I did, and still do, quite a lot of teaching at the Sydney Showground, which is a large agistment/livery centre situated adjacent to Centennial Park in Sydney. Around 1993, whilst instructing at the showground, I started to teach Tim Game, a barrister. Tim simply loved to ride as it gave him a break from his legal commitments, and after teaching him for some time he asked us if we would consider keeping a horse for him at our property that we could work during the week and he could ride at the weekends. It meant that instead of staying in the city to ride, Tim would have a good excuse to get out into the country and we happily agreed to the arrangement. Although the first horse we kept for Tim was nice enough he was really only good for trail riding, so some time later Tim decided to buy a horse which he could ride but, hopefully, would be good enough for me to compete as well. In 1994, along came a horse called Boxster who fitted the bill quite nicely. I took him to intermediate level while Tim continued to come and ride whenever he could. As time went on, Tim and I decided that Boxster would make a better showjumper than eventer because he was so careful over fences, so he went to one of Australia's top showjumpers, George Sanna, and is still going well today showjumping at World Cup level. Meanwhile, Tim bought another horse, this time a mare called Carrera, who I rode a little, and then as she was only three, we decided to put her in foal. Since bringing her back into work she has progressed up the grades and I am now riding her at advanced level. Tim still comes to ride Carrera whenever he can.

Michael Pribular

At around the same time as Tim came on the scene, we were also contacted by Michael Pribular who was very keen to buy some horses for me to ride. After looking for some time, he ended up buying Viper and a little bit later he also bought Jeepster, who would go on to become my Sydney Olympic horse.

Viper

Viper came to us as a 5 year old, having done a little pre-novice eventing. He was quite a hot horse but certainly seemed to be talented, so we felt he was worth taking on. Heath Ryan, who has represented Australia in both eventing and dressage and is now the Australian assistant eventing coach, helped me a lot with Viper's flat work, and together we worked out that he wasn't a horse you could ride for long periods of time as he just got more and more tense. However, if I rode him seven or eight times before his dressage test in very short sessions he seemed to settle down and go much better. This, of course, wasn't always a practical thing to do at a one-day event but at a three-day event, where I had more time, the system of several short sessions did make a difference.

Viper was also quite difficult on cross country as he was very strong, and it took me a long time to work out how to cope with that situation. After riding him in a few events and taking him up to novice level, I discovered that he was controllable to a certain speed, which was around 525–550 metres/minute, but if we went faster it was like hitting a turbo button which I couldn't then turn down. To stay in control I had to jump the whole cross country course at around 550 metres/minute, never letting him go any faster. I tried various bits and did a lot of gallop training at home, but nothing really seemed to work until Vicky Roycroft suggested I try a bit which in 1995 was still quite new on the Australian market, an American gag. I decided to give the new bit a go and took Viper to what I had decided would be his last one-day event, as by this stage it was getting a little scary not being in control as we approached a fence. The difference the American gag made was quite unbelievable. I think because the actual mouthpiece is basically a snaffle, it doesn't really pull the horse's mouth around, but the leverage action of the gag works quite well and consequently it has the desired effect. That's not to say Viper didn't object when I asked him to slow down – he would certainly throw his head around somewhat – but at least I could get him back to safe speed in front of the fence and then allow him to gallop on after jumping it. Once I realised I had that control, I was almost throwing the reins at him in between fences knowing that I would be able to bring him back without too much of a problem. It made the whole cross country experience for both of us less stressful, and as Viper started to enjoy his job he started to jump better. I took him up to advanced level before he was sold to a showjumper, although he went back to eventing with his new owner a few years later.

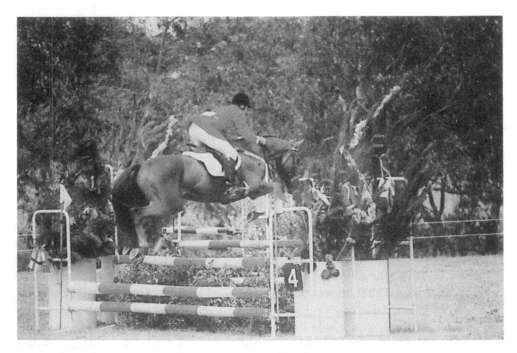

Figure 9.4   The showjumping phase was never a problem for Viper.

Jeepster

Jeepster came to me as a 5 year old. He had done some low-level showjumping with Australian showjumper Chrissy Harris. Chrissy found Jeepster to be quite difficult on the flat, not because he was hot, but because he was quite willful and his reaction when asked to do something tended to be, 'No I don't want to'. Chrissy's husband, Heath, who is a stunt horse trainer, thought Jeepster might become more submissive if he was taught a few 'tricks', including how to bow, lie down and do the Spanish walk. Unfortunately, Jeepster soon learnt he could use these 'tricks' as a way of avoiding doing what I wanted him to, so it took a long time (probably around 3 years) to really learn how to get the best out of him. I worked hard at trying to make his paces bigger so he wouldn't be able to slip back into Spanish movements, but often the minute he felt pressured the Spanish walk would reappear. During those 3 years we could certainly put together some good movements in a dressage test, but there would often be a few threes mixed in with the eights. Jeepster's jumping was never really a problem because, right from the start, he seemed to really love it and jumped whatever I pointed him at. It was his dressage that took the time to get right. We tried to aim Jeepster for the Atlanta Olympics in 1996 but he was simply not yet good enough in the dressage phase. Despite this, his good jumping performance brought him up to finish sixth at Lochinvar CCI***, the Atlanta selection trial, but the selectors had already made the decision to take only the first five riders. Looking back, it probably wasn't a bad thing that we didn't go because, although I felt confident Jeepster would jump the cross country course, I knew his dressage was still inconsistent and could well let him down. In 1997, Jeepster and I were really starting to get our act together and we won Melbourne CCI***. We followed up that the next year by winning Lochinvar CCI*** and were then selected for the 1998 World Equestrian Games to be held in Pratoni, Italy. It was around this time I figured out that if I worked Jeepster for quite a while before his dressage he would usually be quite submissive in his test. Using this method at the World Games put us into a good fourth place at the end of dressage, and we went on to go clear cross country which moved us up to second. Sadly, the showjumping let us down, and after taking two rails down we dropped back to eighth.

After returning to the UK from the World Games, I decided to leave Jeepster, together with Tex who had come over to Europe as my reserve horse, at Jane Bailey's. The plan was to aim both horses for Badminton the following year. While I was still in Australia, Jane brought Jeepster and Tex into work for me in the spring of 1999 and I went back to England just in time to do a couple of warm-up events before Badminton. Unfortunately, at one of those events (Weston Park), Jeepster cracked his stifle and ended up having a year off to recover, so he never made his Badminton debut. Thanks to some great physiotherapy Jeepster made a full recovery and by the spring of 2000 he was back home in Australia, going as well as ever and on track for a place in the Australian team for the Sydney Olympics. Lochinvar was the selection trial for the Olympics and Jeepster proved his good form by coming second and was then shortlisted for Sydney. Thanks to the performances of my other horses (Tex who had come fourth at Lochinvar and Ava who had won Melbourne CCI*** in 2000), I was in the enviable position of being selected for the Sydney team with three horses to choose from, although Jeepster was certainly thought to be the most experienced. By the time Sydney came along, Jeepster and I had really cracked the dressage and it was a great feeling to know that all those years of hard work had paid off at the right time, as we came fourth after dressage on a score of 36. For obvious reasons, the Sydney Olympics will always be very special to me – after all, it's not every day the Olympics are on home territory, and to come away with a team gold medal was just the icing on the cake. Credit for the Sydney result must also go to my team mates: Andrew Hoy and Darien Powers, Phillip Dutton and House Doctor, and Matt Ryan who rode Kibah Sandstone.

After the Olympics, Jeepster was turned out on a well deserved holiday and the following year (2001) I planned to take him to Adelaide CCI****, but half way through his preparation he hit himself in the paddock and got a splint. I gave him a few months off and then brought him back into work, and although he was never really lame he wasn't quite right and we decided to surgically remove the splint and give Adelaide a miss. The following aim was Sydney CCI*** in the early part of 2003 which was a selection trial for the World Equestrian Games, this time to be held in Jerez, Spain. Once again, Jeepster came into work and seemed to be quite sound until the splint started to grow back. This time we kept working him slowly but two weeks before Sydney he was not one hundred per cent so we repeated the splint removal operation and turned him out. Although the splint has returned, it is now much smaller and more settled so hopefully it won't cause a problem in the future. It was a hard decision not to run at Sydney in 2003 because I felt fairly confident I could have got through the event and gone quite well, but sometimes you have to look at the bigger picture. In the back of my mind I see Jeepster as my Athens Olympic horse and that is the most important thing. So Jeepster has had a relatively easy time since

Sydney. I brought him into work later in 2003. He felt really good and one hundred percent sound so we went to Adelaide CCI**** where we came second. Jeepster is certainly giving every indication of being back on track and we hope he will be fighting fit for Athens.

Sue Walker

In 1995 a friend of ours, Sue Walker, an advertising producer, contacted us about her horse Tex. She had been doing dressage with him, but for various reasons had decided to sell him and wondered if we knew anyone who might be interested. Tex had a great personality. He was quite laid back and very easy to work with, and although he had done very little jumping he confidently jumped 1.10 metres and was not at all worried by cross country fences. Because of all these good points we thought we should buy Tex ourselves, but after discussions with Sue we decided to go into partnership, which meant I got the ride on a nice horse and Sue kept her connection with Tex and could still enjoy watching 'her horse' compete.

Tex

Tex was a 6 year old when he came to us and he has always struggled a bit with his flat work, basically because he is a big, long horse. Having said that, he is also a trier, and that's what has made him so good to work with over the years. From the beginning he was good to jump, and after one pre-novice run I took him up to novice, and from then on he never really looked back, getting up to CCI*** level in just one year. As he moved up the grades you could almost guarantee that Tex would finish on his dressage score and in 1998 after coming second at Melbourne CCI*** he was selected as my reserve horse to go to the World Equestrian Games in Pratoni, Italy. I had taken both Jeepster and Tex to the UK, and when Jeepster got on the World Equestrian Games team I decided to take Tex to Boekelo CCI*** in Holland. However, when we got there it rained so much that the organisers chose to turn the CCI into a CIC. Because the going was so bad I did not run Tex at all, so back we came to England. With Jeepster out of Badminton because of his cracked stifle, I decided that Tex was going to be the horse to give me my Badminton debut.

It seemed that from the very start of Badminton the gods were against me, and when, on dressage day, my top boots were actually overflowing with rainwater I should have thought then that something was telling me this wasn't going to be 'my' event. I followed Mark Todd on the draw, which meant I entered the dressage arena as Mark was leaving with the crowd still roaring their approval of his test. Unfortunately, the cheering didn't do a great deal for Tex, who had never seen such crowds and consequently we didn't do the best of tests. Cross country day just went from bad to worse, and from the start of the day I was really questioning whether I should be riding at all in such wet slippery conditions. As I headed off on phase A towards the steeplechase course, I met other riders who were coming back from the chase saying that the track was so muddy and awful they were calling it a day and going home. I remember thinking to myself 'Well that's OK for them, they probably only live a few hours away, but my home's in Australia – I can't just "go home".' And that's the only reason I kept going. Tex coped really well with the heavy ground on the chase course, clocking up one of the fastest times of the afternoon while still picking up 17 time penalties, which just shows how heavy the going was by that stage of the day. The actual cross country course wasn't too bad as the take off and landings of the fences were all-weather, but the going on the flat was pretty treacherous. I found this out when I slipped on the turn after fence five and down we went. I jumped back on Tex and can remember taking the time to think 'Should I keep going?' Looking back, I probably made the wrong decision, but at the time I thought 'What the heck, I'll give it a go.' Things were going really well, with Tex jumping beautifully until we came to the second water. Again the huge crowd around the lake must have looked pretty daunting to my Australian horse. He jumped bravely into the water but really struggled through the lake as the water was above his knees. As we jumped out of the lake and I attempted to keep my balance, Tex kept going on a straight line heading for the most obvious route, which, as he saw it, was a gap in the crowd straight in front of him. Unfortunately, that route was part of the roped-off area, and in actual fact we should have made a very sharp right hand turn as we came out of the lake. Poor Tex didn't really do anything wrong, he just decided that if his rider wasn't telling him anything different he should stay on the most obvious straight line. Luckily, because there was a gap in the crowd, no one was seriously hurt, but at that stage I knew enough was enough and we walked back to the stables. So for me, Badminton was a disaster on two counts: Jeepster never made it there and Tex, through no fault of his own, didn't complete the event. Perhaps one day I'll get back to Badminton, and hopefully second time round will be a happier occasion than the first.

Since 1999, Tex has continued to achieve consistently good performances at all the major three-day events in Australia. At the moment he is being ridden by Husref Malik from Malaysia, who is training with me in preparation for the Athens Olympic Games. Tex is the ideal horse to give someone like Husref experience at the top level, and so far he is going really well.

Kathy Ward and Peter O'Connell

In 1995 I was teaching Kathy Ward at the Sydney Showgrounds, during which time she bought two 3 year old mares, Gifted and Ava. Gifted was a very sweet horse and Kathy really enjoyed riding her, but from the start she found Ava very difficult. Being kept at the Showgrounds where she was stabled for 23 hours a day and only taken out to be ridden didn't help to improve her mind, so Kathy asked us if Ava could move to our yard for some schooling which would also have the added benefit that she could live outside.

Ava

When the diminutive 152.4 cm (15 hh), 3 year old Ava came to live with us, she was so small we never really thought of her as a proper horse, more like something to school and ride around. Although we jumped Ava a little bit, Kathy had bought her as a dressage horse because she had really good movement, so certainly, in the beginning, we stuck mostly to dressage training. Over time, Ava started to grow and when she reached 157.5 cm (15.2 hh) we thought we might have a little play at eventing – nothing serious, but at least it would give her something to do and get her out and about. Ava has always had a certain presence about her and when she was a 4 year year old we took her to the young event-horse class at the Sydney Royal Show, which she won. By the time Ava was a 5 year old she had grown to about 162.6 cm (16 hh). Around this time, Kathy, together with her husband Peter O'Connell, decided that due to her own work commitments she was never really going to have time to work more than one horse so she asked me if I would be interested in eventing Ava more seriously. I think we were all quite surprised when Ava started to show herself to be quite a talented little horse, and went on to compete, at a young age, in several one-day and three-day events. In 1998, as a 6 year old, Ava completed her first CCI** at Adelaide where she finished eighth and the following year she did her first CCI*** at Melbourne, coming ninth. During the 5 years I rode Ava we had some wonderful results, including coming first at Melbourne CCI*** and Spray Farm CIC*** and then second at Adelaide CCI****, all in 2000. She was also shortlisted for the Sydney Olympics, although both Jeepster and Tex had more experience than her, and

Jeepster was the horse which finally ended up getting a run. When I rode Ava at Adelaide in 2000 I ended up showjumping her with one arm in a sling, as a fall from Tex had left me with a broken collar bone. If I had to ride any of my horses with one hand she would be the one to choose because, although she might be a little hot, she is basically good to ride and doesn't pull you around too much. After Adelaide 2000, we decided to give Ava a year off simply because she was still very young at 8 years old and had done quite a lot in a relatively short period of time. I also thought that as 2001 was not a selection year for anything, it seemed a sensible time to give her a break. So during 2001 she had a good holiday and then came in to do some dressage competitions. In 2002 she came back into proper work and went to Sydney CCI***, the selection trial for the World Equestrian Games, and after coming second we headed off to Spain where we enjoyed a really good event until the showjumping phase where we had several rails down. I suppose it was one of those times you would really rather forget, especially when it was so out of character for Ava who is usually such a careful horse. However, simply because of the nature of eventing, you probably have to endure these moments at some point in your career, although I could quite happily live without them!

Ava was always a much better three-day event horse than a one-day horse because the former gave her more time to settle in and get used to her new environment, which helped to produce a much better dressage test. At some one-day events when we attempted to do a dressage test while the cross country was running, it was all I could do to keep her in the arena. Despite this, I really enjoyed riding Ava because she was a lovely, soft, supple horse to train and the package came together with a very switched on brain, which helps to make her such a great cross country horse.

Ava was sold to European rider Susanna Bourdane, and because there are so many events in Europe she is able to compete on a very regular basis, which I'm sure will suit her. At the time of writing, Ava and Susanna have already won a CCI***.

We are still very involved with Kathy, Pete, Tim and Sue, who are all on the look out for other horses for me to ride so that we can do it all again!

My life today

During the years I have been involved with eventing I have been lucky enough to ride some very nice and some not so nice horses, and all of them – even the not so nice ones – have taught me something.

Nowadays, I try to pick the right horse for the job early on. For instance, I might buy a horse which I feel will make a competent novice horse for someone who will probably only ever want to compete up to novice. On the other hand, if I'm looking for something that I hope will turn into an Olympic prospect for myself, I'll look for a slightly different type of horse. Of course, for financial reasons, most of the horses on my yard have to be for sale. At times that can be quite sad, especially when you feel you have a really good horse, but realistically you can't keep all of them. Last year I found myself with three splendid four star horses, Jeepster, Tex and Ava, as well as a very promising three star horse. In Australia, there are simply not enough three star events to warrant keeping more than three top horses, so the last horse was sold overseas. I'm sure she'll go onto become a top horse, just not my top horse.

A typical week's work at the Tinney yard involves Karen and myself riding horses at home, our own and clients', and teaching both at home and around Sydney. The amount of teaching I do depends on the eventing calendar. Obviously, most weekends are taken up with some sort of competition – events, dressage and showjumping days. However, riding, working horses and, indeed, teaching is my job, so I make sure that I balance it with being a fabulous dad to my two daughters Jaymee and Gemma, and a super husband to my ever talented and gorgeous wife Karen!

Stuart's results

Year	Event	Horse
1986	Queensland 3DE Champion CCI**	Radical
1988	5th Queensland 3DE Champion CCI***	Patch of Silver
1988	Trans Tasman 3DE team Championships CCI***	Patch of Silver
1988	Australian 3DE long list for team selection	Patch of Silver
1989	3rd Queensland 3DE Champion CCI***	Patch of Silver
1991	4th Gawler CCI***	BB
1992	2nd Saumur CCI***	BB
1995	4th Gawler CCI***	Viper
1996	1st Berrima 3DE CCI*	Tex
1997	1st Melbourne CCI***	Jeepster
1998	1st Lochinvar CCI***	Jeepster
1998	2nd Melbourne CCI***	Tex
1998	8th World Equestrian Games, Pratoni, Italy	Jeepster
1999	4th Adelaide CCI****	Tex
2000	2nd Lochinvar CCI***	Jeepster
2000	4th Lochinvar CCI***	Tex
2000	1st Melbourne CCI***	Ava
2000	1st Spray Farm CIC***	Ava
2000	Team gold medallist, Sydney Olympic Games	Jeepster
2000	2nd Adelaide CCI****	Ava
2001	9th Melbourne CCI***	Tex
2001	11th Adelaide CCI****	Tex
2002	2nd Sydney CCI***	Ava
2002	16th World Equestrian Games, Jerez, Spain	Ava
2003	2nd Adelaide CCI****	Jeepster

Index